THE
SMILE METHOD

HOW TO
AVOID
GUM SURGERY
AND
DENTURES

Vasilios Gardiakos

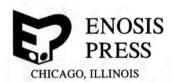

ENOSIS
PRESS
CHICAGO, ILLINOIS

COPYRIGHT 1994 VASILIOS GARDIAKOS

REVISED SECOND EDITION
COPYRIGHT 1997 VASILIOS GARDIAKOS

ISBN 0-9646271-1-6

Library of Congress Catalog Card Number: 97-60553

PRINTED IN U.S.A.

Assistance and advice in writing this book was generously provided by my friends, which I thank with all my heart: Vasiliki Gardiakou (my sister), Gare Unnewehr, Richard Heller, Ann Elgin, Judy Torigoe, George Weiss, Ted Urzedowski, Leigh Kanellakos, Stathis Souladikas. A very special thanks to Helen d'Assatouroff.

I also wish to thank my freinds for all the help provided in preparing the second edition of this book: Michael Jurgaitis, M.D., Paul Nektaredes, John O'heron, Margaret McMullen, Milly Joplin, and Terry Allison. A very special thanks to George Panayote.

*This book is dedicated to my family.
It is through their patience
and sacrifice that I was able to
perform the necessary research
and write this book.*

CONTENTS

INTRODUCTION

There are two reasons why you may want to read this book. One, your dentist has informed you that you have periodontitis, a form of gum disease. He may have recommended gum surgery (or root planing, curettage, antibiotic fibers, tooth extraction or dentures). You value your dental health and are searching for a noninvasive, economical and painless way to stop the disease process and save your teeth.

The second reason is that you are a dentist, periodontist, dental hygienist, dental researcher or educator and want to broaden your knowledge about the treatment of periodontitis. I am confident that this book will benefit both readers, though this book is primarily addressed to the former who has early, moderate or advanced adult periodontitis.

If you have adult periodontitis, here briefly are your choices: If you do nothing, your gum line will recede, your teeth (more than likely healthy, functional and attractive) will loosen and painfully fall out one at a time. Another possibility is that your dentist will extract one or more of your teeth. Granted your dentist can later "replace" your missing teeth with artificial ones such as a bridge, full or partial dentures or implants. However, these expensive replacements are never as good as your natural teeth.

You may elect to have gum surgery which is expensive, painful and disfiguring, or you may choose the nonsurgical techniques detailed in this book that stop the progression of periodontitis. You have nothing to lose and everything to gain by trying the conservative program recommended herein. I will later explain thoroughly why you have nothing to lose and how to painlessly retain your money, health, teeth and smile.

The early history of my dental health was filled with errors. Some were due to my dentist and others were of my own making. These mistakes caused most of my gum health problems.

For many years after my twenties I did not get any additional cavities. I assumed that all was well in my mouth. I figured that my brushing technique and the toothpaste used, was the reason why.

Yes, looking back, there were symptoms of disease, but because I did not have any new cavities, I saw no reason to visit my dentist. My dental visits became irregular. However, the day of reckoning arrived with a vengeance on one of those overdue visits.

In 1981 my family dentist diagnosed me with advanced adult periodontitis. He recommended that I have gum surgery. Though he explained the details of this procedure very calmly, by the time I left his office I felt as if I were handed the death sentence.

I was concerned about the expense, and terrified of the pain. The surgery would expose more of the tooth surface which makes the teeth appear longer. This would make me look older and alter my appearance (for the worse)!

My gut instinct told me not to have surgery performed. Although my dentist did not mention alternatives, deep inside I felt that there must be some. I decided to investigate. With only a little effort I found enough information on nonsurgical treatment of periodontitis to whet my appetite.

I read many dental texts, books and journals on periodontitis, I went to health shows, conventions, and attended many lectures. My studies included all aspects of the disease and especially the alternatives to gum surgery. I was determined to find a way to save my teeth and gums. I did not want to shortchange myself in any way. Much of what I learned I applied and as a result my gum health improved.

On several occasions, I told my dentist about my research. Though he was not aware of some of the treatments and unfamiliar with the others, he dismissed all of them as useless. He insisted that there are no alternatives to gum surgery. After all, if periodontitis can be treated nonsurgically, he would know about it and maybe even prescribe it. If these treatments had even partial success they would be taught in the dental schools.

At each visit he repeated, "Look at the X-rays, you have many pockets, you have bone loss, you have periodontitis. You will lose your teeth unless you have surgery." In the natural progression of this disease the gum detaches from the tooth and forms a pocket. The pocket provides a protected environment where bacteria can thrive. Brushing, flossing and irrigating cannot reach let alone kill the bacteria in the pocket. The bacteria infect the pocket causing it to deepen and destroy more of the underlying bone which supports the teeth. The tooth gradually loosens and eventually falls out.

My dentist ignored my wish to treat my gums without surgery. It seems to me that he wanted to make sure that I had gum surgery performed. He did not differentiate between the active state when the pocket is infected and the state when it is free of infection. When the bacteria is killed the infection is eliminated and the pockets stop getting deeper. The remaining supporting bone is preserved which helps prevent tooth loss.

Five years later my gums were looking and feeling good. Even my dentist noticed the improvement (though he insisted I would still lose my teeth). My symptoms were less frequent and less severe. I went for my biannual oral prophylaxis (teeth cleaning) and examination. What followed was a critical gum infection with abscesses forming on both of my lower first molars.

With much pain I called to see my dentist. I took the systemic antibiotics (capsules) that he prescribed and in a few days I felt better. He offered no hope and made no effort to save my two teeth. He heard my complaints of pain, saw the abscesses and decided to extract both teeth. Though something inside me said "don't", I bowed to the voice of authority and allowed the extractions.

At this point I developed some doubts about the merits of nonsurgical treatment of periodontitis. Many questions came to mind. Could the abscesses have been prevented? Why did I get an abscess following my prophylaxis? If he incised and drained the abscess, how much would that have helped? Could antibiotics have been used more effectively? Why did he choose to extract both teeth? Could my two teeth have been saved by any means? Would gum surgery have saved my two teeth? Should I have gum surgery before I lose any more teeth? How much healthier would my gums be if my dentists had cooperated with me?

Shortly thereafter I found out that my abscesses were caused by what dentists refer to as a "post-prophylaxis periodontal infection". People with periodontitis are prone to such infections because their pockets are full of bacteria. Abrasion or minute cuts are inflicted on the gum during probing, scaling and polishing. Bacteria can more easily penetrate the gum tissue through these openings. This may worsen the infection and form an abscess.

My dentist took no precautions to prevent infection, which can develop as a result of his probing and tooth cleaning. This cost me the loss of my two teeth. Their loss caused additional dental problems and expense. Dear Dentist, if you are reading this... Yes, I have forgiven you... No, I did not have gum surgery as you said I should... Yes, I am still following my method and... No, I have not lost any teeth like you said I would.

My dentist should have taken several precautions to prevent infection. He could have used a subgingival irrigator to apply antiseptics such as a hydrogen peroxide and a saturated salt solution. He could also have used a highly diluted chloramine T. solution into the periodontal pockets after the cleaning. An antibiotic (tetracycline) solution could have been applied in all the high risk or infected pockets (e.g. my two molars). The minimum he should have done is to have provided me with a 1.0% hydrogen peroxide and/or saturated salt warm water solution for me to rinse with.

Still the gut feeling that surgery was not the answer to my gum problems continued. After all, so much of my research pointed in that direction. My desire to avoid the pain, financial, physical and cosmetic persisted.

I decided to expand my research and to look for a new dentist. I asked everyone that I thought may know a dentist that is open to nonsurgical treatment of periodontitis. A friend recommended a dentist which I called and made an appointment to see. This was the turning point. If only I had done this earlier!

This dentist patiently listened to my problems. He was interested enough to hear the details about how I treat my gums. He remarked that what I was doing must be helping as my gums exhibited only a few signs of disease. He respected my choice of treatment and helped me to fully implement it. He was open-minded and always positive. A truly fine person and dentist. His support and encouragement helped me to continue my research and to write this book.

The moral of this story is: if your present dentist recommends that you have gum surgery and does not want to consider a nonsurgical home-care program, then find another dentist and get a second opinion. Preferably, do not obtain the second opinion from a dentist or periodontist that he recommended.

Try to get a second opinion from a dentist that may be considered "holistic", "alternative" or "preventive". Inquire at your local health food store, ask your friends or see the list of organizations listed herein. Look for a dentist who will not create friction and will listen and assist you to treat your periodontitis without surgery as described herein. Find a dentist that has an open mind, is positive and that does not insist that his patients assume a passive role. There are dentists out there who are willing to help you with your goal; so look around. Treat this book as the third opinion.

As it turns out gum surgery does not have such a great track record. Gum surgery does not cure periodontitis. Gum surgery alone does not stop the progression of periodontitis. This is why dentists always recommend that a daily maintenance program be followed after surgery. Too often, even when this lengthy program is complied with, the infection and damage to gum and the underlying supporting bone continues its course. This may require the surgery to be repeated.

I did not know if I could devote the time and handle the cost of up to twenty office visits that surgery requires. The numerous antibiotics, injections, incisions and stitches required and lengthy recovery period that often results was even a bigger concern. I became even more determined not to have it done first time!

I was more encouraged this time around. My success at preventing and eliminating shallow pocket infections had improved. It seems the refinements I made in the diagnostic methods, technique, dentifrice and implements helped my gum health. I also had fewer symptoms and gum infections in my troublesome deep pockets. I was on the right track.

Confucius said, "No doctor is a good doctor who has never been ill himself." Early on when I had setbacks, this idea encouraged me to continue my research. Hippocrates wrote "Physician heal thyself." This principle motivated me to continue until I was completely successful.

My interest in doing this research went beyond the obvious reason, that is, mere direct personal health benefit. The interest to discover first hand, ways to make life healthier, pushed me to do even more research. Lucky for me, I have a talent for research.

Physicians and researchers, in the past, often used their bodies to experiment and test the effectiveness of their treatments. In light of this tradition, to broaden my understanding of periodontitis and to save my teeth I became my own guinea pig. I often neglected my gums so that the bacteria will multiply and promote infection. These infections gave me the opportunity to experiment and improve the various techniques. My method had to prevent and eliminate all infections regardless if they were in shallow or deep pockets, even if abscessed.

The research entailed many experiments that were done without the pressure of meeting a specific deadline. The results were time tested in a natural setting. I applied the time honored Hippocratic scientific principles of keen observation of patient (and guinea pig), record keeping of symptoms and diagnosis. Over the fifteen years of research, this helped enormously in formulating and refining the procedures that kill the bacteria and eliminate the gum infections due to periodontitis.

Necessity, the mother of invention, inspired me to develop the means to apply natural antiseptics to the base of deep pockets. I named this instrument VITAPICK (previously HAPPICK and MICROPICK). This practical deep pocket applicator gave me the means to reach and kill the destructive bacteria in all my pockets deeper than 4mm. The VITAPICK allows me to eliminate and prevent infections in my deepest pockets in the comfort of my home.

If only I had the VITAPICK years earlier, I would have been able to prevent or eliminate the abscesses that formed in pockets 10 to 12 millimeters (1/2"). This was the missing ingredient that made my method fully effective. With this final innovation I could control all aspects of the disease process and save my remaining teeth and gums.

The reason you do not see D.D.S. after my name is that I am not a dentist. I have no professional ties or obligations. As a researcher this independence gave me the flexibility to study all health disciplines and philosophies. When I began this research I had no bias or preconceived notions how to treat periodontitis. I started with a clean slate and freely searched anywhere and everywhere.

Dentists often look outside their profession for fresh ideas and inspiration. As a group they are open to new and better ways to care for their patients. I hope they find the concepts recommended herein worthwhile and incorporate them into their practice.

Satisfied patients that maintain healthy gums without surgery will tell their family, friends and neighbors. For the dentist, healthier patients will reduce stress, and hopefully provide greater financial independence. This may be a simplistic way of looking at the advantages, but what is important is that everyone wins!

My main concern is how the financially and politically powerful dental institutions will react to this book. Will they feel threatened by it? Will they try to undermine my efforts to inform the public about their periodontal options? Will they ignore me in the hope that I will somehow vanish? Will they help spread the message? Stay in contact for the outcome.

Newton wrote that he could see further because he stood on the shoulders of the giants of ancient Greece. I can see far because I stand on the shoulders of those giants of medicine and the tall dental researchers of the last two centuries. Without their ingenuity, dedication and inspiration I would have lost some teeth or even become toothless, rather than writing a book about saving them. I am very grateful to them, for they risked so much when they shook the foundation of their respective great institutions.

My research incorporates ideas from the AMERICAN DENTAL ASSOCIATION through and including the AMERICAN NATURAL HYGIENE SOCIETY. Much was borrowed from Dr. Paul Keyes and the INTERNATIONAL DENTAL HEALTH FOUNDATION which he co-founded. I used the holistic approach which utilized the best parts from each of these diverse health disciplines.

The scope of this book is to inform you of what is safe and practical to use. It is a comprehensive step by step "what to", "when to", and "how to" reference guide, organized to be as easy to use as 1, 2, 3. A few "why" questions are briefly answered for the sake of causality and continuity. I devoted some space to the theories on the causes and progression of periodontitis, because I feel this will help clarify and unite all the concepts. For the dental researcher and for those who have the time and interest, I included many references used in my research and to which I am heavily indebted.

Knowing that most people are busy, I have kept this book to the point. For smoother and faster reading, I have avoided citing references in the formal notation as used in medical books and journals. For the same reason I have limited the use of direct quotations. I know there are many female dentists, but in order to help the book flow, I refrained from using the "he/she" or other nonspecific gender expressions in favor of the traditional "he".

Some methods for treating periodontitis have been with us for a long time, many are current. I combined the old and new practices, modified and refined them and employed all that modern technology has to offer. I perfected some tools and techniques and added the insight of my personal experience and that of others.

To make things practical, I eliminated time-consuming tasks and shortened and simplified others. As the saying goes, in science and medicine and as well in everyday life, if you want something to work, "Keep it simple." For a sneak preview of how simple it is, turn to section 14.

I followed the Hippocratic principle of nonmaleficence; first do no harm. There are many chemicals that will destroy the pathogens that cause gum infections but unfortunately they may also harm the patient (and the guinea pig). For this reason I carefully selected ingredients that were tested and proven safe to use. In formulating the antiseptic solutions used in the VITAPICK, for brushing and all the other tasks, I used FDA (Food and Drug Administration) approved drugs, USP (United States Pharmacopoeia) items, orthomolecular substances (items that the body naturally and normally utilizes) and/or edible and consumable ingredients. I also include in the second edition, colloidal silver, the leading antiseptic prior to the development of antibiotics.

I developed safe and simple procedures to apply prescription and nonprescription antibiotics in the gum crevice and pockets. The application of antibiotics locally, enhances their effectiveness, while requiring only one thousandth of the amount that is often prescribed to be taken orally. This eliminates the many side effects that usually accompany systemic antibiotics.

I have personally tested and am presently using all that is described in this book. Some of my pockets are over 10mm deep with severe bone loss, yet my teeth are white, fully functional. My gums are firm and healthy looking. I no longer get gum abscesses. My breath is fresh. I have not lost any teeth, which is better than the three to five that I may have lost if I had done nothing to improve my gum health. Most of the time I practice periodic preventive care. When occasionally I slack off and symptoms return I follow my advice which quickly returns my gum health and prevents further damage.

The cure for periodontitis, it seems, is a long way off. Fortunately, you can now kill the destructive bacteria in the deepest pockets and improve your gum health. You can avoid gum surgery and save your teeth. This is the reason I named it THE SMILE METHOD. I hope it will put a SMILE on your face.

During the last few years that this book and the applicator were available, many users, dentists and other health professionals informed me of the success that they had following THE SMILE METHOD. I thank them for their testimonials and support. I hope that this updated book and applicator reaches and spares many more people from the invasive periodontal procedures practiced by modern dentistry.

PART I
GUM DISEASE

1. DEFINING DISEASES OF THE GUMS

In this book, for the most part, I will use language that the average person can understand. I am limiting the use of medical terminology mostly Greek and Latin polysyllabic tongue twisters (no... tongue twisting does not cause periodontitis!).

(1) **Gum disease** and periodontal disease are terms that describe all gum afflictions though lately they are sometimes used interchangeably with periodontitis.

(2) **Gingivitis** (both g's as in ginger) is an infection and inflammation of the gum tissue. The underlying supporting bone is not affected. Trench mouth, Vincent's infection and acute necrotizing ulcerative gingivitis (A.N.U.G.) are various forms of gingivitis.

(3) **Periodontitis** (adult periodontitis, pyorrhea) the most common of all adult gum disorders and the main focus of this book is a chronic debilitating disease. In the active state, bacteria infect and deepen the gum crevice and form a pocket. This infection is also the primary mechanism which erodes the underlying bone that supports the teeth and gums.

2. PERIODONTITIS FORMS POCKETS

Periodontitis causes the deepening of the gum crevice (crevice or groove but properly called gingival crevice or sulcus) that surrounds each tooth. This leads to the formation of pockets (properly called periodontal pockets). Your dentist can easily locate and fairly accurately measure crevice and pocket depths.

(1) Why and how the crevice deepens is not a well understood process. The crevice may deepen in the weakest or most susceptible sites or areas of greatest or persistent irritation. The crevice between the teeth is more susceptible due to the fact that the toothbrush cannot reach there.

(2) Bacteria accumulate in the deepened gum crevice which may cause **inflection**. Infection then further deepens the crevice.

(3) At some sites around the tooth, infection in the crevice further detaches the gum from the tooth. This forms a pocket (very crudely resembling a shirt pocket).

(4) The **major complication of periodontitis** is when pockets deepen to more than 4 mm.

    (a) Deep pockets provide a protected environment for the bacteria that cause infection. Brushing, irrigating, flossing and swashing **do not reach the base** of deep pockets. These tasks help to some degree to prevent deep pocket infections but are useless to eliminate them. To eliminate and prevent reinfection a deep pocket applicator like the VITAPICK must be used to deliver antimicrobial solutions to the base of the pocket.

    (b) Deep pockets are more likely than shallow pockets to be infected and have severe prolonged infection and abscess formation.

    (c) In deep pockets there is no correlation between pocket depth and frequency and severity of infection. In other words your 10 mm pocket is not more prone to infection than your 6 mm pocket.

(5) Pockets are permanent. There is no way to reattach the gum to the tooth though after eliminating the infection a minor reduction of pocket depth may occur.

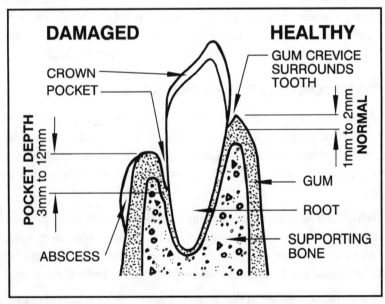

CROSS-SECTION OF A TOOTH

3. PERIODONTITIS CAUSES BONE LOSS

Persistent and recurring infection in the gum crevice and pockets slowly destroys the bone that supports the gum and teeth. Duration and severity of infection determines how much bone is lost (dissolved, resorbed). The destruction is irreversible. There is a close correlation between pocket depth and bone loss. Usually the deeper the pocket is, the greater is the bone loss. You can detect bone loss but only your dentist can determine how much has been lost.

(1) Bone loss leads to loose teeth. You can see or feel the loose tooth by holding it between two fingers, and for more accuracy hold the tooth against the fingernails and wiggle.

(2) Bone loss may cause teeth to migrate or drift apart making the space between teeth grow wider. When chewing, the opposing teeth can jam food particles in the space and in the pocket. You may find yourself probing with your tongue or using a toothpick more often. Dislodging the food particles from between the teeth and from the pocket will become increasingly more difficult. Food particles packed in the pocket increase the risk of infection. Ask your dentist about reducing the space between the teeth.

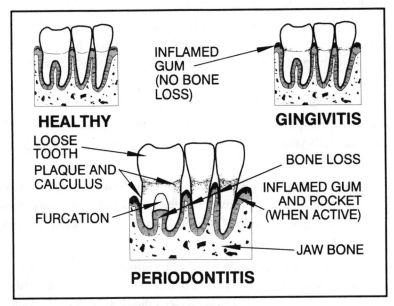

GINGIVITIS AND PERIODONTITIS

(3) As you lose the bone that shapes the gum, the gum line recedes, exposing more of the tooth. Visually this and tooth migration is more noticeable on your front teeth.

(4) As the gum further recedes it exposes the root which is yellowish. This is not insulated by enamel thus the nerves that are inside your teeth are more easily effected by stimuli. You may have an increased tooth sensitivity to hot or cold liquids or even an increased sensitivity to hydrogen peroxide and/or salt solutions used for brushing.

(5) Bone loss may change how your dentures fit and how your opposing teeth meet when they come together.

4. PERIODONTITIS CAN CAUSE TOOTH LOSS

If periodontitis is not properly treated the infection continues to erode the bone that supports the gum and teeth. Periodontitis causes 70% of all adult tooth loss (30% from tooth decay). Periodontitis does not damage the teeth, so those lost due to this disease are often healthy and functional.

(1) If you do not treat your periodontitis, **your teeth will fall out one at a time**. Studies show that untreated periodontitis costs Americans one tooth loss every 2.8 to 4 years. That is five to seven teeth lost over a 20 year period, eight to twelve teeth lost in 33 years! One in eleven Americans over the age of 45 have none of their natural teeth left.

(2) If your gum health has deteriorated so much that your teeth fall out, this may mean that you have lost so much supporting bone that dentures may not be properly fitted. Once the decision is made in favor of dentures, extract the teeth and thus conserve the supporting bone. Seek advice from your dentist.

(3) If you cannot keep a tooth free from infection, due to inaccessibility (more likely your third molars), then consider extraction. Ask your dentist for advice.

(4) All missing teeth (other than third molars) **must be replaced** with artificial dentition to avert future problems. Your dentist can advise you on restorations; full or partial dentures, fixed or removable bridges and tooth implants.

(5) Very loose teeth may be immobilized if splinted to adjacent firm teeth. This may be a practical alternative to tooth extraction. Your dentist should make sure that you will be able to feed the floss under the splint.

(6) Your dentist may recommend extracting very loose teeth. **Do not** consent to tooth extraction until you have been following THE SMILE METHOD for at least one month. By then you will know to some degree how much your gum health has improved. Often "hopeless" teeth can be saved.

5. CLASSIFICATION OF GUM DISEASE

Damage done by periodontitis varies throughout the mouth, so that some sites are healthy while others may be at various stages of disease. This makes classification of periodontitis difficult. Your dentist can classify the status of your periodontitis, though he may use a different index or different method of classification than the one outlined below. The list below should be used only as a rough guide.

(1) **Type I- Gingivitis** - no bone loss, no loose teeth, pockets under 4 mm (due to gum inflammation rather than gum detachment).

(2) **Type II- Early Periodontitis** - a little bone loss, no loose teeth, pockets 3-6 mm deep.

(3) **Type III- Moderate Periodontitis** - moderate bone loss, a little tooth looseness, pockets 5-8 mm deep.

(4) **Type IV- Advanced Periodontitis** - substantial bone loss, pronounced tooth looseness, pockets over 7 mm deep.

(5) **Type V- Refractory Progressive Periodontitis** - continued gum infection with bone destruction in spite of treatment.

(6) APPROXIMATE EQUIVALENTS: 3 mm = 1/8", 6 mm = 1/4", 9 mm = 3/8", 12 mm = 1/2".

6. SYMPTOMS OF ACTIVE PERIODONTITIS

A **symptom** is an observed or sensed physical deviation from the normal which may indicate disease. **Active** means that a harmful infection is present. Often when the gum is infected, symptoms are manifested. Keep in mind though that in early and sometimes moderate periodontitis, symptoms may be minor, hardly noticeable or non-existent. Chronic low grade gum infections also may not exhibit any obvious signs. Often there is no pain and this is the main reason most people do not visit their dentist. Infected gums may exhibit none, some or all the symptoms listed below.

(1) **Bleeding** is one of the best indicators of a gum infection. Tiny ulcers (open wounds) are formed in the gum crevice and pockets during infection. These ulcers can bleed easily. Gums may bleed when brushing teeth, irrigating, flossing, when using a toothpick, when using the VITAPICK or when massaging gums, chewing or even spontaneously.

    (a) Blood may be easily visible on the toothbrush, floss, saliva or in the overflow from your mouth when irrigating or rinsing.

    (b) Bleeding may be very slight and confined within the crevice. It can only be seen by close examination. A dental mirror, along with a very well lit cosmetic mirror may be used to inspect (prior to rinsing your mouth). To check for minor bleeding you may rub or press a cotton swab across the gum line and inspect it for signs of blood.

(2) **Pus** in the gum crevice is a sure sign of infection. You may be able to see, smell, taste or feel it with your tongue.

    (a) A clear exudate though harder to detect than pus, is also a sign of infection. Pus is white but if mixed with blood it may be pink.

    (b) When irrigating the stream may force out some of the pus which may give off an offensive odor. Smell the floss. A foul odor, it may indicate infection.

    (c) You can maneuver your tongue or press with your finger to squeeze out the pus. Avoid swallowing the pus and clear exudate. Rinse mouth.

(3) A periodontal **abscess** can be acute (quickly forming) or chronic (slowly progressing). An abscess always indicates infection.

    (a) Usually an abscess may be seen or felt as a bump on the gum.

    (b) Often it is warm and painful.

    (c) Sometimes it may be sensed by shaking or tapping the head, or by the impact of walking or running.

(4) There may be slight **discomfort** or pain due to inflammation which increases the pressure that is exerted on the nerves. Inflammation forces the tooth slightly out of the socket. This may become noticeable when chewing because the affected tooth prematurely contacts the opposing teeth. To test this, clench your teeth and try to feel this discrepancy.

(5) You may have **bad breath** (halitosis), especially that fetid odor of decay and disease. Bad breath due to gingivitis or infected gum due to periodontitis can range from mild to very offensive. Bad breath is not an absolute symptom of gum infection. Do not confuse it with bad breath due to other causes.

 (a) Clasp hands over nose and mouth and exhale. Carefully inhale through your nose and monitor your breath odor. Alternate exhaling and inhaling several times. Check your breath odor often at first until breath odor improves, and at least weekly thereafter.

 (b) Another method is to get a small new plastic bag (the kind used for storing food) and blow in it from your mouth. Then slowly squeeze the bag while sniffing the exhaust.

 (c) If you can not tell if your own breath is foul, ask a family member, friend, your dental hygienist or dentist to take a sniff and give you an honest opinion about its odor. If they survive, there is hope!

 (d) By trial and error you will eventually be able to distinguish between bad breath odor due to gum infection and other causes. Bad breath may result from many health problems, improper digestion, odorous food and beverages consumed, poor dental hygiene or the presence of dental cavities.

(6) Red, swollen, spongy, inflamed, sore, tender, stinging, discomfort, pain and hypersensitive teeth, are signs of possible infection. The presence of plaque and calculus do not indicate infection.

7. PATHOGENS AND PERIODONTITIS

Though there are many theories, the **cause** of periodontitis is not known. What causes the initial damage and deepening of the crevice is not addressed herein as it is especially full of controversy. Research has generated many facts about gum infections, yet this has not helped our understanding of what causes periodontitis. When the crevice is damaged, the gum, it seems, becomes susceptible to infection. The focus here will be on infections in the crevice that has already deepened and pockets that have formed.

(1) Normally the bacteria that inhabit all parts of the mouth **promote health.**

(a) Most if not all of the bacteria that is thought to cause infection is present in the flora but in an ecological balance without causing disease.

(b) Pasteur may have correctly stated, "The presence in the body of a "pathogenic agent" is not necessarily synonymous with infectious disease." He is reported to have said when late in his years, "...the seed is nothing, the soil is everything." Are the "offending" bacteria found in the crevice or pocket the cause of disease or the result of it?

(2) There have been many studies to determine which bacteria **promote periodontitis**. A diseased pocket has tiny open wounds or ulcers. That is why the pocket may bleed when probed or sting when a hydrogen peroxide or salt solution is delivered into it. The elimination of the "offending" bacteria allows the tissue to heal. I will not name any of the suspected culprits but will use the more general terms, "plaque", or "bacteria" or the more descriptive "periodontopathogens" (sorry about the tongue twister) or "pathogens".

(a) No single bacteria has been isolated and conclusively implicated. None of the suspected bacteria has fulfilled Koch's postulates, a set of conditions that if met would prove causality.

(b) Certain bacteria are never found or are present in very small numbers in a healthy gum crevice but are often found in large quantities in infected sites.

(c) Some of the many bacteria that normally or occasionally reside in your mouth under the proper circumstances interact and participate in promoting disease.

(d) Researchers are fairly certain that some of the gram-negative, anaerobic bacteria below the gum line in large quantities promote infection. Some of the bacteria found above the gum line may to a lesser degree also be responsible.

(e) It is not certain if all gum infections deepen the pockets and destroy the supporting bone. It is also not certain how bacteria or their toxic by-products cause damage.

(3) **Plaque** is an organized sticky film composed of saliva, loose epithelial cells, debris and over 300 forms of bacteria. The prevalent view today

is that it is in this form that bacteria can promote infection. Note though that the presence of plaque does not indicate infection.

(a) Plaque reorganizes and colonizes within 24 hours after it has been disrupted.

(b) As the plaque forms in the gum crevice and pockets, the bacteria at some point begin to cause damage. It is sometime during this active state that most of the permanent damage to bone and gum occurs.

(c) Plaque is invisible to the naked eye but when it accumulates it becomes translucent, off white, greyish or yellowish. Teeth that normally feel smooth or polished to the tongue, may feel rough when there is plaque buildup.

(d) The plaque that accumulates above the gum line does not share all characteristics with plaque found below.

(e) Plaque can easily be disrupted, loosened or partially removed from the tooth mechanically (and chemically) by brushing, irrigating and flossing. In deep pockets the VITAPICK with the proper solution chemically kills the bacteria.

(4) **Calculus** (or tartar) is a coarse inert deposit on the surface of teeth. Its presence does not indicate infection.

(a) Calculus is formed when dead bacteria accumulates, mineralizes and hardens.

(b) Calculus can also be formed without the presence of plaque. It can be formed by the accumulation of mineral salts found in saliva. This type of calculus may more readily be found on the inside lower front teeth and the outside surface of the upper molars which are near the salivary ducts.

(c) Depending on how it formed and its composition calculus may be yellowish, brown, black, orange or green.

(d) What makes the calculus undesirable is that it is coarse and porous which can house bacteria. The bacteria can reside and multiply out of the grasp of the brush and floss though not out of the reach of antiseptic and antibiotic solutions. Calculus may act as a mechanical irritant though its detrimental effects, if any, have not been demonstrated.

    (e)   Calculus can only be removed with the use of a scaler. It can not be removed by brushing or flossing.

(5) Periodontitis is **probably not contagious**.

    (a)   It has never been demonstrated that non-resident bacteria cause or promote periodontitis.

    (b)   It is unlikely that periodontopathogens are transmittable from person to person by kissing or other means in sufficient quantities to cause disease. Lowered resistance to infection due to poor health and a host of other conditions must be present for this bacteria to contribute to the disease process. If your gums are not susceptible you will not be affected.

    (c)   Periodontal infections usually return within a short time. Infections recur maybe because the pathogenic bacteria is never completely eliminated. It may be that the conditions that promote infection have not improved.

    (d)   Some sites may go into remission or into a long period of quiescence which does not support that periodontitis is contagious. It is also unlikely that an infected site can contaminate a healthy one.

(6) Periodontitis may be one of the few infectious diseases that is being treated without ever identifying the specific pathogen or pathogens.

    (a)   The theory that bacteria **causes** periodontitis rests on a shaky foundation.

    (b)   The disease-bacteria-infection-disease model as the main mechanism by which pockets deepen and the underlying supporting bone is destroyed, is used herein primarily because it is a fairly consistent concept which can be used effectively to stop the disease process.

    (c)   Antiseptics and antibiotics are used because they stop the disease process at least temporarily. The cycle is broken and then you see improvement of gum health and the elimination of symptoms.

8. OTHER FACTORS IMPLICATED IN PERIODONTITIS

It is likely that periodontitis has multiple causes. Some factors that may cause or promote periodontitis are listed below.

(1) If **gingivitis** is left untreated, it can lead to the more severe periodontitis. This may be due to inflammation which forms a "pseudo" pocket where periodontopathogens can multiply.

(2) **Smoking** and chewing tobacco besides being detrimental to overall health, also stain the teeth. Stained, dirty and yellowish teeth or the lack of hygienic care may contribute to periodontitis. Pathogens more easily accumulate on stained teeth.

(3) Refined or **white sugar** (sucrose) consumption contributes to dental, bodily and mental ill health.

    (a) We know that bacteria flourish when refined sugar is present in the mouth.

    (b) Refined sugar consumption may increase calcium secretion which weakens the jaw bone.

    (c) White sugar consumption suppresses the immune system.

    (d) The complex sugar, fructose found in fresh ripe fruits are good for health though to a lesser degree, they too can promote bacterial growth.

(4) Due to receding gum line **cooked food** can be impacted in the crevice or pocket, especially between widely spaced teeth. This may irritate the gum and cause infection. This will then further recede the gum line. The chewing action when eating most raw fruits, vegetables and nuts cleans the teeth which reduces plaque accumulation. If lodged between teeth, they do not easily ferment.

(5) Improper brushing or using **stiff toothbrushes** can damage the healthy shallow gum crevice. This may start the cycle of disease.

(6) **Snapping of floss** when inserting it or "digging" into the crevice with too great of force when flossing can injure the healthy gum tissue.

(7) Toothpicks, especially splintered **wood toothpicks** may pierce the gum and introduce pathogens into the tissue.

(8) Caps (crowns), inlays and fillings (amalgams) with **overhangs and ledges** may cause food particles, debris and plaque to accumulate. These anomalies make removal of the accumulated debris and hygiene difficult. You may notice that the floss shreds or gets snagged by the overhang or ledge. See diagram in section 66(5).

(9) **Malocclusion** or poorly aligned opposing teeth and clenching or grinding of teeth may retard healing and thus promote periodontitis.

(10) **Xerostomia** (dry mouth or cotton mouth) is the reduction or absence of saliva in the mouth. Saliva promotes oral health with its antiseptic, and tooth recalcifying properties. The absence of saliva can facilitate periodontitis and other health problems. Some of the causes of dry mouth are:

(a) Prescription and over the counter drugs and radiation therapy.

(b) Alcohol consumption and cigarette smoking.

(c) Sjogren's Syndrome, diabetes, hypertension and Parkinson's disease.

(d) Mouth breathing instead of breathing through the nose.

(e) Fever, stress, depression, nervousness and fear.

(f) Not rinsing mouth after taking sodium ascorbate (and possibly other forms of vitamin C) in solution. Inadequate rinsing after brushing with salt solution or baking soda may also contribute.

(11) People with a family record of periodontitis may be predisposed to get it. This predisposition could be due to **genetics** but more likely is the result of a shared environment and life-style **disease producing habits.**

(12) Some **medications** and oral contraceptives can be hazardous to gum health. Steroids, some types of anti-epilepsy drugs, cancer therapy drugs, some calcium channel blockers may also contribute. Broad spectrum antibiotics taken systemically may disrupt the natural flora thus allow infection to take hold. Ask your dentist if any drugs you may be taking are affecting your gums.

(13) **Low vitamin C level** in the serum but more important low tissue level may predispose one to gum problems.

(14) There may also be non-infectious means by which bone is lost such as dietary deficiencies and diseases like osteoporosis. **Vitamin and mineral deficiencies** that adversely effect the bone may be implicated. Eliminating dietary deficiencies may help to slow down the disease process but no evidence exists that the disease can be reversed.

(15) Dental carries (cavities, tooth decay) do not cause periodontitis though they have overlapping etiological factors.

9. WHO IS SUSCEPTIBLE TO PERIODONTITIS

The prevalence of gum disease worldwide is at epidemic levels. Over 95% of Americans either have or will suffer from some form of gum disease during their lifetime. Thirty two million people in the U.S. are afflicted with advanced periodontitis. Early and moderate periodontitis are even more common.

(1) 75% of Americans over 35 years old have periodontitis, though many younger Americans also have it. In fact periodontitis may start at an early age and be first diagnosed much later. Aging and old age do not cause periodontitis but the years of wear, tear and neglect of the oral cavity and bad eating habits and diet eventually catch up to most of us.

(2) People who never brush or floss, eat the standard American diet (SAD), do not exercise and have disease producing habits are more susceptible to periodontitis. Yes, there are people in this group that do not have cavities or periodontitis. These people are the exception.

(3) Diabetes does not cause periodontitis but it facilitates it. Diabetics have a high incidence of periodontitis due to the susceptibility for infection and delayed healing.

(4) AIDS does not cause periodontitis but it may facilitate it. Periodontitis often is one of the first symptoms of AIDS.

(5) Osteoporosis does not cause periodontitis. Though periodontitis does not cause osteoporosis, it may precede osteoporosis by 10 years. The loss of bone mass of the jaw often is an early sign of osteoporosis and periodontitis.

(6) People with thyroid disease are at a higher risk to periodontitis.

(7) Women are more susceptible to periodontitis than men. This may be so for the same reason that women are more prone to osteoporosis. Their thinner more delicate bone structure makes them more vulnerable, because they have less bone to "sacrifice" to disease. During menstruation often some symptoms similar to periodontitis appear. If untreated it can lead to periodontitis.

(8) Pregnant women may get symptoms of periodontitis which often go away after childbirth. Women should be extremely careful in how they deal with these symptoms or treat their periodontitis, because whatever they do may hurt their fetus.

10. PREVENTING PERIODONTITIS

Though there is much controversy on the initial cause of periodontitis, much can be said about the factors that prevent it. Following are some ideas on prevention.

(1) Proper diet and life-style can improve your chances of not suffering from periodontitis.

    (a) We know that people who live on raw fruits, vegetables and nuts have a much lower incidence of periodontitis. This is also true of "primitive" societies consuming their native diets exclusively, even without brushing or flossing! When their progeny consume the "modern" diet they fall victim to periodontitis.

    (b) Dental researchers should spend more time investigating why these groups have such healthy mouths instead of why we have so many dental problems.

(2) Healthy, energetic people are less likely to have periodontitis. There are many ways to promote physical health, some are better than others. See section 98, HOW TO IMPROVE YOUR HEALTH.

(3) People who do most of what their dentist tells them to do, have healthier mouths than people that do not. I am sure there are people reading this thinking, "I saw my dentist often and did everything (everything?) he told me to do and I have a bad case of periodontitis." There are even more people that say, "I never saw a dentist (I wish I had) and look I have periodontitis!"

(4) One may hypothesize that since THE SMILE METHOD can prevent periodontitis from progressing, it may also stop it and gingivitis from developing. The routine for prevention need not be as thorough nor include the use of the VITAPICK deep pocket applicator.

11. PERIODONTITIS AND HEALTH

There is a relationship between the health of your gums and your general well-being. As you improve the health of your gums, this correlation will become more clear to you.

(1) Hippocrates wrote, "The human body is like a circle, any point may be considered as both the beginning and the end... by the affection of one part, the next will also suffer." This holistic concept that if your gums

are infected, you will feel weakness in your body and if your body is ill, then your gums will be more susceptible to infection is true but not always obvious because of the time lag between cause and effect.

(2) Your energy level may be low and you may feel run down when your gums are infected.

(3) An abscess that is draining pus into your mouth can lead to "cold" symptoms, sore throat and decrease appetite due to the foul taste in your mouth. If a periodontal or periapical abscess has formed, the pressure caused by the chewing action when eating can force bacteria into the blood stream. If this infection spreads systemically, fever may result.

(4) Advanced periodontitis can make proper chewing more difficult.

    (a) This may be due to chewing inefficiency from loose or missing teeth. An infected site may increase discomfort, which usually leads to reduced mastication which then adversely effects digestion.

    (b) We do not often think about it but an important step in proper digestion is having a healthy mouth. The food goes through certain "preparation" in the mouth before reaching the stomach. We may say then that digestion actually begins in the mouth. Taking care of your gums and teeth is an important step in having proper digestion. To go a step further, proper digestion means better overall health.

(5) Advanced periodontitis with much bone loss can cause teeth to shift. Shifting molars may cause headaches, pain in the neck and jaw hinge and cause ears to ring. The shifting teeth cause improper alignment of opposing teeth which decreases chewing efficiency.

(6) THE SMILE METHOD can help your general well-being by eliminating the health burden caused by gum infections. There is suspicion that bacteria in the crevice and pockets feed sinus and gastic ulcer infections. You must take care of the part that is ill, so the whole body will not suffer.

PART II
THE PLAN

12. ADVANCES PROMOTED BY THE SMILE METHOD

THE SMILE METHOD, has broken new ground in many areas in the conservative nonsurgical treatment of early, moderate and advanced adult periodontitis. Briefly, some are listed below.

(1)   The grouping of periodontal pockets into shallow and deep, each with a preferred treatment method.

(2)   The use of the VITAPICK applicator to kill bacteria in deep pockets. This can prevent and eliminate infections and abscess formation in deep pockets.

(3)   The use of safe, effective and economical antiseptic solutions to quickly kill the destructive bacteria and eliminate gum infections.

(4)   The use of highly diluted 35% food grade hydrogen peroxide as an antiseptic.

(5)   The use of the U-TIP, that makes irrigating gums and teeth safer, faster and more effective at treating shallow pocket infections.

(6)   Unique, accurate and easy to perform diagnostic procedures.

(7)   Unique method used to stop bleeding gums with floss.

(8)   The use of vitamin C, mega and C-NBT doses.

(9)   Unique, safe procedures to apply prescription and nonprescription antibiotics locally, at home.

(10) Swashing, a unique way to use the one antiseptic mouthwash that you always carry with you; saliva.

13. THE SMILE METHOD - PROS AND CONS

Below is a list of what THE SMILE METHOD is, what it can and what it can not do for you, if you have adult periodontitis.

(1)   It can not cure periodontitis. Like gum surgery it cannot reattach the

gum to the tooth nor reverse the damage to the underlying supporting bone.

(2) THE SMILE METHOD can stabilize your gum health. It focuses on diagnosing, treating and preventing infections in the gum crevice, shallow and the hard to reach deep pockets.

   (a) If you follow it, you will have fewer if any gum infections, the main mechanism by which gum and bone are damaged. This may make some pockets shallower, firm up the gum and strengthen and save loose teeth.

   (b) THE SMILE METHOD can also help prevent your gum line from receding further, whiten and brighten dull stained teeth, improve breath odor, and promote health in general.

(3) It is easy to implement.

   (a) Just read this book and follow instructions. THE SMILE METHOD will be easy to follow since you are probably familiar with most of the tasks and may be routinely performing some of them already. The new tasks are fairly easy to learn.

   (b) THE SMILE METHOD is a **dentist-assisted** program. If your dentist is not familiar with THE SMILE METHOD he can assist you to implement it by following the NTD guide. See section 25.

   (c) THE SMILE METHOD can also be a **dentist-managed** program. If a dentist is familiar with THE SMILE METHOD he will tend to all aspects of the program. He will motivate, instruct, train and assist you to implement it. He will monitor your progress and modulate (adjust) the treatment as needed.

(4) It is not very time consuming. THE SMILE METHOD daily routine may take less time to perform than the routine prescribed by your dentist or periodontist after gum surgery. It may take only a little more time than what most people with healthy gums spend to brush and floss their teeth. The bedtime program which includes brushing the teeth, gums and tongue, irrigating and flossing with practice can be done in as little as five minutes! See section 14 and 15.

(5) It is painless to perform the various tasks.

(6) It is relatively inexpensive to follow. The daily expenses are low and dental visits are minimized. Remember that part of the cost of eating and drinking should also include keeping your gums and teeth healthy.

(a)   The VITAPICK, electric-brush, irrigator, , FLOXITE lighted mirror, dental mirror, and the lip and cheek retractor cost under $200 (in 1997 dollars). If amortized over two years it comes out to 28 cents per day (over four years at 14 cents per day!).

(b)   The use of manual-brushes, the consumption of floss, hydrogen peroxide, baking soda, salt and ten grams of vitamin C daily, costs approximately 52 cents per day.

(c)   Not including visits to your dentist your grand total expenses comes out to less than 80 cents per day! The money saved with THE SMILE METHOD can be used on dental prosthetics (for loose and missing teeth), dental cosmetics, or a vacation. It is your money, spend it wisely.

(7)   You have nothing to lose by implementing THE SMILE METHOD.

(a)   Gum surgery and root planing are not emergency procedures. This allows you time to improve your gum health with this conservative method first. Later you can decide in favor or against gum surgery and root planing (or extraction and dentures).

(b)   While following THE SMILE METHOD you may still elect to have gum surgery performed. The surgery may not be as extensive and healing and recovery will be accelerated. After surgery slowly integrate THE SMILE METHOD while your gums are healing.

(8)   For THE SMILE METHOD to work, it must be followed. If you stop following THE SMILE METHOD, the symptoms and hence the infections will return and cause additional damage to your gums and bone.

14. THE SMILE METHOD - OUTLINE

Dr. Turner, a long-standing expert on periodontitis, states "There is no such thing as a periodontal disease, there is a spectrum of disease." There may be no single procedure to treat periodontitis, hence THE SMILE METHOD uses a multifaceted approach. The various tasks attack periodontitis systemically, topically, locally (primarily in the pocket), mechanically and chemically, internally and externally. THE SMILE METHOD routine tasks listed below should be performed periodically as noted. Tasks in bold are part of THE SMILE METHOD daily routine.

(1)   Periodically visit your dentist for oral prophylaxis, examination, diag-

nosis and to assess the pocket depth and bone loss status. See PART III -YOUR DENTIST.

(2) **Manual-brush your teeth in the morning with soda and electric-brush at night, preferably during the bedtime program. Use a salt (and hydrogen peroxide if needed) warm water solution.** See PART VI - BRUSHING.

(3) **If you choose to irrigate, it is best performed during the bedtime program. Add salt (and hydrogen peroxide if needed) to the warm water in reservoir.** See PART VII - IRRIGATING.

(4) **Floss preferably during the bedtime program.** See PART VIII - FLOSSING.

(5) **Be on the alert for symptoms of infection.** See section 6, SYMPTOMS OF ACTIVE PERIODONTITIS.

(6) **Take vitamin C.** See PART XIII - SUPPLEMENTS.

(7) **Swash at least three times per day.** See PART XII - SWASHING.

(8) For preventative purposes every three to fourteen days use the VITAPICK applicator on all deep pockets or at minimum all troublesome pockets. Apply hydrogen peroxide and salt solution. See section 74(3).

(9) Perform diagnostics on suspect and troublesome sites often and promptly when a site exhibits symptoms. See section 17, DIAGNOSTICS - HOW YOU CAN DIAGNOSE A GUM INFECTION.

(10) Treat suspect and diagnosed gum infections accordingly. See PART XI -TREATING GUM INFECTIONS.

(11) Occasionally review this book to make sure that you are doing everything properly. Refine your routine to maximize its effectiveness.

15. THE BEDTIME PROGRAM

Add the bedtime program to your established nighttime "list of things to do" which may include showering, setting the alarm clock, setting the thermostat, stretching and watching T.V. Perform the bedtime program nightly and you will awaken in the morning with healthier gums and a fresher breath. The tasks listed below should be performed in the order listed.

(1) **Electric-brush** with a salt (and hydrogen peroxide if needed) solution. Swish the leftover solution vigorously in mouth.

(2) **Irrigate** with a salt (and hydrogen peroxide if needed) solution. Swish the leftover solution vigorously in mouth. Skip irrigating if your deep pockets do not improve or infections worsen.

(3) **Floss** after brushing or after irrigating.

(4) When finished brushing, irrigating and flossing, manual-brush your tongue then **rinse** your mouth thoroughly with warm water.

(5) No food or beverage should be consumed during the interval before sleeping.

   (a) If you take cough syrup, chewable or liquid anti-acids during this time, depending on the substance it may be best to brush again or rinse your mouth with water.

   (b) Water, pills, vitamin supplements, capsules and vitamin C solutions may be consumed without the need to brush again.

(6) The other possible task that you may want to include (daily, occasionally or when necessary) as part of THE SMILE METHOD bedtime program are:

   (a) Take vitamin C.

   (b) Massage gums with fingers.

   (c) Perform diagnostics.

   (d) Use the VITAPICK to prevent or eliminate gum infections.

   (e) Treat suspect and diagnosed gum infections.

16. THE THREE PHASES OF THE SMILE METHOD

The primary goal of THE SMILE METHOD is to stabilize your periodontitis, so that no additional damage occurs. This is accomplished by preventing or shortening the duration of infections in the gum crevice and pockets. Using this three phase system simplifies this process.

(1) **DIAGNOSIS** - Through symptom recognition and periodic diagnosis locate infected pockets and determine if they are shallow or deep. See section 14(1), (5) and (9).

(2) **TREATMENT** - Follow procedures to eliminate suspect and diagnosed shallow and deep pocket infections. See section 14(10).

(3) **PREVENTION** - Most of THE SMILE METHOD tasks are formulated to maintain gum health, by preventing reinfection. See section 14(1)

through (8) and (11).

(4)   Simply put: Monitor your gum health daily, follow the daily routine to maintain gum health and diagnose and treat gum infections. In the simplest terms when you are following THE SMILE METHOD, you are mostly preventing and if required eliminating gum infections.

17. DIAGNOSTICS - HOW YOU CAN DIAGNOSE A GUM INFECTION

Knowing or at least suspecting which sites are infected is essential for treatment. It is important to perform diagnostics regularly and to locate and treat gum infections promptly. Unfortunately, there is no fool proof method to diagnose if a pocket is healthy or if it is infected. Dentist and self diagnosis are the weakest link in the treatment of periodontitis.

(1)   Low grade gum infections that are asymptomatic are difficult to locate and diagnose. Gums may look healthy when they are not. You may diagnose infection when a site is healthy. Often your diagnosis will be inconclusive. One consolation is that low grade infections cause less damage, though if left untreated the damage will accumulate.

(2)   You should always be on the alert for symptoms. An analysis of symptoms will aid you in a proper diagnosis.

   (a)   To be on the safe side, assume that at the location of every symptom is an infection (especially near deep pockets).

   (b)   You should at regular intervals record the symptoms for a comparative analysis so that you may modulate the routine to optimize your gum health.

   (c)   To test the accuracy of your diagnosis ask your dentist for his opinion, which sites are infected.

(3)   Dentists use the indicator, "bleeding upon probing" (see section 29(3)) as strong evidence that a pocket is infected. You can get similar results by using the VITAPICK applicator. See section 74(3).

   (a)   Fill the applicator with hydrogen peroxide and salt solution.

   (b)   Insert the tip in the pocket and eject solution. See section 66.

   (c)   If a pocket bleeds when inserting the tip, the pocket is probably infected. You may see the blood as it overflows from the pocket.

   (d)   On suspect or troublesome sites if the bleeding is not obvious, you may check for minor bleeding by rubbing a cotton swab along the front and back gum line. You may also use the dental mirror to spot minor bleeding in areas out of direct sight.

(4) When irrigating gums or using the VITAPICK applicator with salt solution and/or hydrogen peroxide and a stinging, burning or numbing sensation in the gum crevice or pocket may occur. This very sensitive indicator usually signals that an infection is present.

   (a) When using the VITAPICK, stinging may be the first sign of infection to appear and the last to go away when it clears. Once periodontitis has been controlled this diagnostic tool is the best one to use as it is capable of alerting you even to low-grade infections. See section 74(3).

   (b) Though it may be quite painful in severe infections, it usually is not. The pain or discomfort lasts only a short time. The stinging will be reduced as the infection is diminished. Be thankful that you are being warned! To minimize stinging, use the VITAPICK to apply the equivalent of a drop or two of solution to the base of the pocket. You may use a more dilute solution which stings less.

   (c) Stinging is more frequent in the crevice or pocket under a faulty cap. The stinging here may be due to either an irritated raw or infected gum. See section 90 and diagram near 66(5).

   (d) Minor stinging may be due to irritation caused by the insertion of the tip. What may feel like stinging or burning may be the result of tooth hypersensitivity and not infection. See section 96.

   (e) You may not sense any stinging if the tip of the VITAPICK and hence the solution do not reach the site of the infection at the base of the pocket.

(5) Look for pus (milky, yellow or pink) around a problem site that you suspect is infected. Press finger, cotton swab or dental mirror on the gum to see if any pus oozes out. The presence of pus always indicates infection.

(6) With one finger or thumb apply pressure (a little more than chewing pressure) on the chewing surface of each tooth. Bite on a wooden chopstick to test one site at a time and note the sensation. The teeth that hurt while applying pressure may be infected.

(7) Use the periodontal probe, or metal spoon and **lightly** tap one tooth at a

time on the front surface and mentally note the sound. **Be careful not to chip your teeth!**

   (a) The odd sounding teeth may confirm an infection or may indicate sites where the greatest bone loss has occurred.

   (b) Next, tap on the chewing surface of teeth and notice the sensation. Percussion may cause discomfort or pain on the tooth of the infected site. However, note that pain does not always indicate infection.

(8) At least once monthly, and prior to using the VITAPICK, massage the gums. Use your index finger or thumb and massage the outer and inner, lower and upper gums and roof of mouth. Use short strokes and medium amount of pressure.

   (a) Note where on your gum you feel any discomfort or pain due to the applied pressure. Compare the sensation with nearby healthy gum which is firm.

   (b) Check gum for softness or a spongy sensation which may indicate an infection or an abscess.

   (c) Where the gum is inflamed or there is a bump there often is infection or an abscess. Inflammation may also be caused by trauma and other means.

(9) Check under chin and along the jawbone for inflammation. Swollen glands may indicate gum infection (or other health problems). "Walk" your thumbs under the chin and along the jawbone, apply a little pressure and try to sense irregularities and discomfort.

(10) Dark red, bluish red and especially bright red gums may indicate infection. Touch the gum to see if it quickly returns to its normal color. If it does not, it may be due to infection.

(11) SUMMARY: Any of the following signs may indicate gum infection: Red, swollen, spongy, inflamed, sore, tender, blood, stinging, discomfort, pain, hypersensitive teeth, bad odor or taste, plaque and calculus. Pus and abscess always indicate that a site is infected.

18. POCKET PENETRATION BY VARIOUS MEANS

To control your periodontitis, it helps to know the **maximum** penetration and effectiveness of the various tasks.

(1) **Mouthwash and Lozenges** - 1 mm (1/32") - may dislodge and destroy some plaque above the gum line.

(2) **Swashing** - 1 mm (1/32") - may dislodge and destroy some plaque above the gum line.

(3) **Brushing** - 2 mm (1/16") - very effective at removing plaque mechanically above the gum line and a little below but ineffective between the teeth. Antiseptic dentifrices increase effectiveness.

(4) **Tea Tree Oil** - 3 mm (1/8") - has good penetrating and antimicrobial capability when applied directly on dry gum. Do not use if it irritates the gum.

(5) **Irrigating** - 4 mm (1/8"+) - Dental irrigators are very good at removing food particles and loose plaque and delivery of antiseptic solutions in the gum crevice but not in pockets.

(6) **Flossing** - 4 mm (1/8"+) - very effective at disrupting or removing plaque from the crevice, below and above the gum line but only between the teeth. When antiseptics or antibiotics are added, it is good at treating infections in the gum crevice. Floss cannot reach into pockets.

(7) **VITAPICK** - 12 mm (1/2") - the only way to apply antiseptics and antibiotics in deep pockets at home. By using this applicator you will be able to diagnose, eliminate and prevent deep pocket infections.

19. STARTING THE SMILE METHOD

When first starting out and until you become familiar with THE SMILE METHOD follow it very carefully. You will find that it is fairly easy to follow, if you take one step at a time.

(1) Purchase all the inspection tools, appliances and consumables as described in the next three sections.

    (a) All of these items may be bought at your local grocery store, health food store, drug store, discount center or by mail order.

    (b) If you cannot locate the VITAPICK and the lip and cheek retractor locally call or write to:

    ALBRITE INC.
    P.O. Box 1095
    Crystal Beach, FL 34681
    813/781-5111   800/533-1821
    email: info@albrite.com website: http://www.albrite.com

(2) Read and save all the manuals, operating and usage instructions, guarantees and receipts at some convenient location for easy referral.

(3) Keep in mind when taking up new habits they will at first be cumbersome and take up more time.

 (a) At first refer to this book often for all the details. I would estimate that within two to four weeks, you will have your treatment program down to the minimum time.

 (b) First perform the tasks correctly. Once perfected, you may try to do them faster.

 (c) Later when you are more familiar with the routine and its results you may tailor it to fit your health needs, life style, time schedule and preferences.

(4) If your gums are in a very deteriorated condition and bleed spontaneously, are swollen, in pain, or have an abscess, implement THE SMILE METHOD in the following manner:

 (a) Start taking C-NBT dosage immediately. See sections 84 and 85.

 (b) Brush, irrigate and floss more carefully and gently at first, so not to irritate the infected sites.

 (c) Consider using the VITAPICK with an antibiotic solution. See section 74(4).

 (d) Slowly implement all aspects of THE SMILE METHOD.

(5) The following is a simple and easy way to help eliminate superficial gum infections. Do this for a week or two or on occasion.

 (a) Add one or two tablespoon salt in a cup of very warm water. Swish the solution in mouth and let it flow between the teeth (left, right then center) up to 5 times per day. Hold the solution near the problem site. Salt solution is anti-inflammatory and antiseptic.

 (b) If you prefer a hydrogen peroxide solution just add 40 to 80 drops of 35% food grade hydrogen peroxide to a cup of warm water (which will yield a 0.35% to 0.7% solution). If this irritates your mouth use a more dilute solution or decrease frequency.

 (c) Alternate using these solutions or add hydrogen peroxide to the salt solution to make it more potent.

(6) If your gum infection has spread systemically (to the rest of your body) and you have fever, you should see your dentist.

(a) Ask him to first consider applying an antibiotic solution in the gum crevice and pockets. See section 74(4).

(b) He may prescribe systemic antibiotics (which you should take). Continue your C-NBT dosage as it will compliment the antibiotic.

(c) He may recommend extracting the "offending" tooth. Consent only if the antibiotics and THE SMILE METHOD fail to eliminate the gum infection or the tooth is ready to fall out on its own.

20. INSPECTION TOOLS - PURCHASING

Using the proper tools listed below will facilitate inspection of your mouth for the diagnosis and treatment of your periodontitis. See section 19(1).

(1) A **dental mirror** with a handle, similar to what your dentist uses to inspect inside your mouth is essential in seeing the tongue side of your teeth and gums.

(a) There are several metal and plastic dental mirrors available locally usually at drugstores.

(b) FLOXITE makes the DETAIL REFLECTOR, a spoon sized magnifying mirror designed especially for self examination. It's plastic and not as clear as a glass mirror, but because of its size and ease of use, I still recommend that you try it.

(c) The MIROLITE by BUTLER and the LUMIDENT by NOAH is a 1" mouth mirror with a small flashlight that projects light to the site to be observed. It is a little bulky, but I still recommend that you try it, especially if you do not have a well lit mirror.

(d) If the mirror fogging is a nuisance, lick the mirror surface to clear the moisture. Better yet, dip the mirror in warm water or run warm water over it to bring it up to your body temperature. This will prevent the mirror from fogging.

(2) I highly recommend a well lit cosmetic mirror or the **FLOXITE** high-intensity lamp with magnifying mirror. The FLOXITE will project light into your mouth which makes viewing and maneuvering of instruments much easier. Most washroom and many cosmetic mirrors are inadequately lit and do not concentrate the light into the mouth where it is needed. Before investing on the FLOXITE see how well you can see in

your mouth with the mirror that you have. If you mount on wall, mirror should be at mouth level.

(3) I very highly recommend getting a **lip and cheek retractor**. This clear plastic device gently spreads your lips and holds your cheeks away from your teeth greatly increasing visibility. This also frees both hands allowing better accessibility. The retractor will save you time.

(4) The **periodontal probe** is a hand-held instrument with a metallic tip that has twelve or more single millimeter markings. If it is color coded, it will make measuring easier.

    (a) The tip is inserted in the gum crevice and used to locate pockets, to measure pocket depth and to see which sites bleed. It is very difficult to measure pocket depth alone or with an untrained help-er, so you may hold off buying this item.

    (b) You can however use it to measure tooth exposure, which is fairly easy to do alone. See section 100(3) and PERIODONTAL PROBE diagram.

(5) Get **cotton swabs** which may be used to rub on gum line to check for blood.

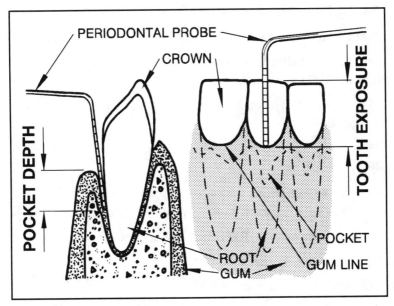

PERIODONTAL PROBE

(6) Many dentists recommend the use of disclosing tablets which, when chewed, stain the plaque that reveal the areas of your teeth that you missed during brushing. It is not certain that the disclosing tablets reveal the plaque that causes periodontitis. The plaque that promotes disease in pockets are not stained nor could it be seen if it was in any case.

21. APPLIANCES REQUIRED - OUTLINE

Below is a list of appliances (implements) required to follow THE SMILE METHOD. To save on shelf space the base units of most of these may be mounted on the wall. See section 19(1).

(1) Manual-brushes (three brands - very soft). See section 52.

(2) Electric-brush. See section 53.

(3) Irrigator (WATER PIK). See sections 56(3) and 58.

(4) VITAPICK (preferably two units). See section 64(1).

(5) Interdental brushes if required. See section 48(2).

22. CONSUMABLES REQUIRED - OUTLINE

Below is a list of consumable items and dispensers required to implement THE SMILE METHOD. See section 19(1).

(1) Baking soda in box or jar. (8 or 16 ounce box is best). See section 37(1).

(2) Salt (plain or iodized) in dispenser. You may substitute Epsom salt. See sections 37(2) and 44(3).

(3) 35% food grade hydrogen peroxide in small drop-dispenser bottle. See section 40(1).

(4) 35% food grade hydrogen peroxide in plastic pint bottle. See section 40(1).

(5) One ounce clear plastic measuring cup that can also measure fractions of an ounce, tablespoon, teaspoon, and milliliters. See section 42(4).

(6) Floss, thin, unwaxed (BUTLER,). See section 60.

(7) Vitamin C. See section 87.

(8) Colloidal silver. See section 37(4).

(9) Tetracycline or equivalent antibiotic if required. See section 67.

PART III
YOUR DENTIST

23. FINDING A DENTIST

Your dentist and periodontist can be your best allies and partners in the treatment of periodontitis (and other oral health problems). Find a dentist that is patient and that will answer all your questions to your satisfaction in a manner that you can understand. Find a dentist that respects your choice of treatment and that will either manage or assist you to implement THE SMILE METHOD.

Some of the organizations listed below will mail you a list of their membership (free or for a small fee) which is composed of health practitioners of which a few or all are dentists. Some of these dentists may practice nonsurgical treatment of periodontitis or may be receptive to new ideas. Some of these organizations publish interesting and informative journals or newsletters. All are located in the U.S.A.

(1) THE AMERICAN ACADEMY OF PERIODONTOLOGY
     737 North Michigan Avenue
     Suite 800
     Chicago, IL 60611
     312/787-5518   website: http://www.perio.org

     They do not have a list of dentists or periodontists that may treat periodontitis without surgery. If you decide to have gum surgery or want more information on surgery call or write and ask them for pamphlets.

(2) AMERICAN DENTAL ASSOCIATION
     211 East Chicago Avenue
     Chicago, IL 60611
     312/440-2500 800/621-8099
     email: SANSONEC@ADA.ORG   website: http://www.ada.org/

     They do not have a list of dentists or periodontists that may treat periodontitis without surgery. If you decide to have gum surgery or want more information on surgery call or write and ask them for pamphlets.

(3) THE AMERICAN NATURAL HYGIENE SOCIETY, INC.
P.O. Box 30630
11816 Racetrack Road
Tampa, FL 33630-0129
813/855-6607   fax: 813/855-8052
email: anhs@anhs.org   website: http://www.anhs.org

(4) DENTAL AMALGAM MERCURY SYNDROME
6025 Osuna Blvd. NE
Suite B
Albuquerque, NM 87109
505/888-0111   Fax: 505/888-0111   email: pbrake@ccsi.com

They have a list of dentists that practice mercury free dentistry. Some may also treat periodontitis without surgery. To order the information and dentist referral packet for a small donation, call 800-311-6265.

(5) INTERNATIONAL ACADEMY OF NUTRITION
AND PREVENTIVE MEDICINE
P.O. Box 18433
Asheville, NC 28814
704/258-3243

They have a list of several dentists that use vitamin C therapeutically.

(6) INTERNATIONAL DENTAL HEALTH FOUNDATION
11160-F South Lakes Drive
Suite 345
Reston, VA 22091
703/860-9244   Fax: 703/860-92445   email: IDHF@aol.com

(7) Inquire at your local health food store or check your local health periodicals and Yellow Pages. You may also check local and national health directories such as The Alternative Medicine Yellow Pages and the New Age Journal Guide to Holistic Health. The Internet is another source to try.

(8) Ask your family and friends.

24. BEFORE YOUR DENTAL VISIT

Before you visit your dentist a small amount of preparation will make it more rewarding.

(1)   Make a list before going to see your dentist.

    (a)   Write down your symptoms. See section 6.

    (b)   Write down which sites you have diagnosed as being infected. See section 17.

    (c)   Write down any questions that you may have regarding your dental health.

    (d)   Date and keep a copy of the list for future referral.

(2)   Copy the NTD (Note To Dentist) and familiarize yourself with it. Bring it along and refer to it or give the copy to your dentist. The NTD is located in section 25.

(3)   Gather all your records, notes, lists, X-rays and charts to bring with you. Review this book and dental terminology. Mentally organize your visit.

(4)   Take C-NBT to help stave off any infection due to the dentist's probing. See section 84.

(5)   Avoid eating odorous food before seeing your dentist. Just prior to your visit, brush your teeth and tongue, irrigate and floss for hygienic reasons and so that your dentist will see a clean mouth.

(6)   Prepare to be on time for your appointment and if you have to cancel inform your dentist as soon as possible.

25. HOW YOUR DENTIST CAN ASSIST YOU

THE SMILE METHOD can be either dentist-managed or dentist-assisted. If it is **dentist-managed**, your dentist will tend to all aspects and details of THE SMILE METHOD and motivate, instruct and assist you to implement it, monitor your progress and modulate the treatment if needed. If it is **dentist-assisted** (your dentist is not familiar with THE SMILE METHOD) then you must ask him to perform the items listed below. This is the minimum your dentist must do to assist you so that you can properly implement THE SMILE METHOD. These items can be properly performed only by your dentist.

(1)   During your initial visit, ask your dentist to do the following:

    (a)   Inform you if you have adult periodontitis and if so, is it early, moderate or advanced. See section 5.

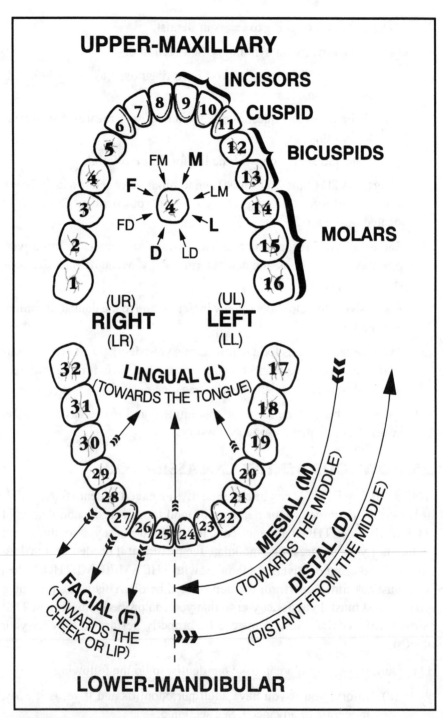

TOOTH DESIGNATIONS

I am following THE SMILE METHOD which is a dentist-assisted home-care program for periodontitis. Your assistance will help me implement it, make it more effective and easier to follow. Please assist me with the following:

(1) Do I have adult periodontitis?

(2) Is it early, moderate or advanced?

(3) Probe pocket depth around each tooth at **six points** and mark on chart.

(4) Point out the location of all my deep pockets (over 4 mm deep) while the periodontal probe is inserted. Please use the lip and cheek retractor to increase my visibility.

(5) Put a **"B"** on my dental chart, indicating all sites that bleed upon probing.

(6) Mark all pockets with an **"A"** (active) that you diagnose as being infected. Write **"P"** where pus is present.

(7) Record tooth mobility on chart (use the Mobility Index).

(8) Provide a 0.5% to 1.0% hydrogen peroxide warm water mouth rinse.

(9) Show me how to properly brush, irrigate and floss.

(10) At the end of my visit apply an antiseptic solution at the base of all my deep pockets with a subgingival irrigator or applicator.

(11) If some pockets bleed upon probing, pus flows, are infected or abscessed, and you feel it is appropriate, please perform the following:

    (a) Prepare an antibiotic solution (probably 40 mg tetracycline per ml of water).

    (b) Apply this solution using a subgingival applicator to the base of all the affected pockets with **minimal overflow**.

    (c) Blot the overflow and remove the visible antibiotic with a gauze pad.

    (d) Advise if the antibiotic application should be repeated.

(12) Give me a copy of the dental chart and your notes.

NTD

(b) Note all the pocket locations and depths on a tooth chart. This will help you to group your pockets as **shallow (4 mm or less)** and **deep (more than 4 mm)**. See section 28(2).

(c) Note which pockets are infected. See section 29.

(d) All the above items are listed on the NTD.

(2) During your initial visit and periodically thereafter, have an oral pro-phylaxis (professional teeth cleaning). See section 27.

(3) It is important to gauge long term progress.

(a) Have your dentist check and record the depth of your pockets every 6 months at first and at <u>maximum</u> every 24 months thereaf-ter if your gums have been mostly free of infection. See sections 28(2) and 100(1).

(b) He should periodically examine to see if any additional bone has been lost. See sections 28(4) and 100(2).

(4) You may need a prescription for antibiotics (probably tetracycline cap-sules) to treat infected or abscessed pockets with floss or the VITAPI-CK. See section 67(2).

(5) If you have overhangs or ledges where your floss gets snagged or shreds, ask your dentist to eliminate them, if it is economically and technically feasible. See sections 8(8) and 90 and diagram near 66(5).

26. DURING YOUR DENTAL VISIT

If your dentist will not manage but you want him to assist you to implement THE SMILE METHOD, note the following:

(1) Relax! Don't be nervous! You are the master of your oral health prefer-ences. If you have chosen THE SMILE METHOD there will be little or no pain. Hopefully you have prepared for this visit as recommended in section 24.

(2) There are an increasing number of dentists that are against gum surgery. However, do not be surprised if your dentist is opposed to your choice of treatment. He may either be uninformed or misinformed about non-surgical treatment of periodontitis.

(3) During your dental visit or perhaps during an oral prophylaxis, you may want to inform your dentist of your choice of treatment.

(a) The NTD may be given to your dentist or dental hygienist to explain what needs to be done so that they can assist you to implement THE SMILE METHOD. This request should not create any problem or conflict since what you are asking your dentist to do is not overly time consuming or difficult to do.

(b) Most dentists routinely perform many of the items listed. See items 1,2,3,5,6,7 and 9 in NTD which are in bold.

(c) To make sure nothing is overlooked check off each item that he performs .

(d) If they seem receptive tell them about or lend them this book.

(4) Some dentists may find getting the NTD upsetting. If you suspect this of your dentist, then do not hand him the NTD but verbalize the contents. Give specific instructions of what you want done. You must take charge of your dental health and "have it your way". Hopefully this will be with consultation, advice and assistance from a supportive dentist. A little diplomacy, a smile and a "please" can help you achieve your goal.

(5) Inform your dentist (and again remind him before surgery or extraction) if you had rheumatic fever, rheumatic heart disease, organic valvular defects, organic murmurs, artificial heart prosthesis, carditis or Sydenham's chorea. For a free pamphlet "Dental Care for Adults with Heart Disease", write to (enclose a business size self-addressed stamped envelope):

THE AMERICAN HEART ASSOCIATION
Box AHM
7320 Greenville Ave.
Dallas, TX 75231
800-242-8721   website: http://www.americanheart.org

27. ORAL PROPHYLAXIS

THE SMILE METHOD routine includes a periodic visit to your dentist for an oral prophylaxis (teeth cleaning).

(1) Scaling is performed by your dentist or dental hygienist during a routine oral prophylaxis.

(a) Calculus may form in areas that you have consecutively missed with the toothbrush and floss. Ask on which teeth calculus has accumulated so that you may correct your brushing and flossing technique.

(b) Scaling the teeth is an effective way to reduce the bacteria in the crevice. Ultrasonic or hand scaling are the only ways to remove the calculus that has accumulated. Scaling may remove calculus as much as 2 mm (1/16") below the gum line.

(c) As a precaution, to help prevent a gum infection, ask to be provided an antiseptic mouth rinse. A warm water 0.5% to 1.0% hydrogen peroxide solution is a good choice. Plain water is inadequate for the final mouth rinse.

(d) The CAVI-MED and ODONTOSON ultrasonic scalers have the capability while scaling to simultaneously deliver an antiseptic solution to the gum crevice. This helps prevent gum infection due to scaling.

(e) Rinse often and look for blood which may indicate a minor cut. Infected gums bleed more easily when probed and scaled.

(f) Every 6 to 12 months (not to exceed 24 months) you should have your teeth professionally scaled. Seek your dentist's advice as to how often. Have your teeth polished only to remove visible surface stains.

(2) Ask your dentist or dental hygienist to use a subgingival applicator or the VITAPICK. This is the best way to reduce the risk of infection from minor cuts that are inflicted on the gum from scaling and polishing.

(a) A 0.5% to 1.0% hydrogen peroxide and saturated salt solution or a very well diluted (less than 1%) chloramine T. (sodium paratoluene sulfonchloramide) solution should be applied to all your pockets, especially your deep pockets, before, during and especially after cleaning your teeth. If stinging is intense, use a more dilute solution until the infection is reduced. See section 74(3).

(b) The pockets that bled during scaling or probing or are diagnosed as being infected may have an antibiotic (probably 40 mg tetracycline per milliliter of water) solution applied into them. Apply only a minute amount to the base of the pocket to minimize the overflow. See section 74(4).

28. HOW YOUR DENTIST CAN DIAGNOSE PERIODONTITIS

A thorough examination and an accurate and detailed diagnosis of your gum health is important for proper treatment. Your dentist will classify if your periodontitis is early, moderate or advanced. It is important that your dentist periodically compare notes from previous visits and inform you if any additional damage has occurred. Your dentist will use more than one of the following diagnostic methods to estimate how much damage has been done.

(1) Your **symptoms** are one of the most important ways for your dentist to diagnose periodontitis. Discuss your symptoms with him. Test the accuracy of your diagnosis, by comparing it with your dentist's.

(2) By using a periodontal **probe**, your dentist will measure the depth of your periodontal pockets.

  (a) He should record on a chart the depth of your gum crevice and all the pockets at **six points** around each tooth.

  (b) Ask your dentist to point to all your deep (over 4 mm deep) pockets, so as to make locating and treatment of those pockets easier at home. You may put a red dot on your dental chart near where deep pockets are located.

  (c) Inserting the periodontal probe in the pocket is generally not painful. To get an accurate reading some pressure is applied momentarily which may cause a little discomfort.

  (d) The periodontal probe should be sterilized between measurements or at least between teeth with a 1.0% hydrogen peroxide and/or saturated salt solution or HIBICLENS to avoid cross contamination. This will not be necessary if the dentist later applies antiseptics or antibiotics in the crevice and pockets.

  (e) Pocket depth measurements, because no proper standards have been established, are not consistent nor very accurate and should be used only as a rough guide. An inflamed gum surrounding a pocket will cause a measurement to read deeper. When the inflammation subsides it will read shallower. A receding gum line without a proportionate deepening of pocket will result in a shallower reading.

  (f) Periodontitis if not properly treated, is a chronic and usually slow progressing disease. Pocket depths change very slowly. Comparing pocket depths is used strictly, as a long term gauge to determine if the disease has stabilized or is still progressing.

(3) Ask your dentist also to determine the **mobility** (the degree of looseness) of each tooth. Your dentist will wiggle each tooth with instruments or fingers and make an estimate of mobility. Using the Mobility Index as a guide he will write the corresponding Roman numeral on your chart.

    (a) Healthy teeth move slightly but are not classified.

    (b) **Class I** - a little more movement than normal.

    (c) **Class II** - tooth movement over 1 mm (1/32").

    (d) **Class III** - in addition to 1 mm movement tooth can also be rotated and pushed in.

(4) The **X-rays** show the present condition of the teeth and the underlying supporting bone.

    (a) A comparative evaluation to determine bone loss is very difficult with X-rays when the loss is minor. It often takes one to three years for the loss to be discernible using X-rays.

    (b) By using digital imaging technology your dentist can measure bone loss or gain in a period as short as four months. This helps enormously to determine the effectiveness of treatment.

    (c) Unless there are other considerations, X-rays for periodontitis should be taken only for comparative purposes.

(5) **CAUTION:** Note the following regarding X-rays:

    (a) Over exposure to X-rays is detrimental to your health so avoid repeat exposure for two years. Ask your dentist to protect you with a thyroid shield during exposure.

    (b) Pregnant women should schedule elective X-rays during second trimester or beyond.

    (c) Ask for E-speed or faster film to reduce X-ray exposure.

    (d) Radiovisiography (RVG), a new digital imaging technology requires only 10% of normal X-ray exposure time.

(6) Healthy gums range in **color** from coral pink, dark blue/purple to brown. Hues vary from individual to individual. Mottled pigmentation of var-

ious dark hues may be considered normal in some individuals. Using a dental mirror, your dentist will also check the tongue side of your gums for coloration.

(7) Healthy gums are **stippled** (pitted or have an orange peel like surface texture). Lack of stippling and smooth and shiny gums may indicate disease.

(8) Your dentist may **photograph** your teeth and gums. An old Chinese proverb says, "A picture is worth a thousand words." If you plan to photograph your teeth at home, use the lip and cheek retractor to increase the amount of teeth visible. Comparing photos from your past with your present condition, can help you determine the effectiveness of your gum care. Though this is only used as a long term gauge it may help motivate you to continue THE SMILE METHOD.

29. HOW YOUR DENTIST CAN DIAGNOSE GUM INFECTION

Diagnosing gum infections is an art not a science. Unfortunately, at present, there is no way to absolutely and positively diagnose active periodontitis or determine if a site is infected (active) or is free of infection (inactive, quiescent). To complicate matters some dentists do not differentiate between the two states.

(1) Tell your dentist which sites have **symptoms** of infection to help him locate the affected sites. If you have diagnosed any site to be infected, discuss your findings with him. To test the accuracy of your diagnosis compare it with your dentist's.

(2) Your dentist's **visual and tactile** inspection of your gum line, teeth, roof of mouth and face can often assist him in locating gum infection and abscesses.

(3) Your dentist will insert the periodontal **probe** to measure the depth of your pockets and to check for bleeding. "Bleeding upon (gentle) probing" usually indicates that a site is infected.

(4) Your dentist may **press gum** with probe or finger to see if the gum is firm and if pus flows out. The presence of pus always indicates an infection.

(5) Contrary to what some dentists may say, gum infections cannot be re-

vealed with **X-rays**. An abscess though, if it's between the teeth in an advanced stage may be discerned.

30. DIAGNOSTIC TESTS

The diagnostic tests below are available for use by dentists only.

(1) The PERIOTEMP and the PERIO-ANALYZER can measure the temperature of pocket. Higher temperatures relative to the norm may indicate infection.

(2) BIO TECHNICA'S DMDX test for periodontitis uses paper points that are inserted into the pockets and later analyzed for pathogens.

(3) The newest test by XYTRONYX and PERIOCHECK by ADVANCED CLINICAL TECHNOLOGIES, INC. will detect the presence of the enzymes that may determine if your gums are infected.

(4) The ORAL-B PERIOSCAN TEST, and the COLGATE PERIOGARD may be used to help in diagnosis.

(5) JOHNSON & JOHNSON makers of PATHOTEK claim that this product can help establish an accurate prognosis.

(6) A dentist properly trained in the Keyes Technique or MMPT (Microbiologically Modulated Periodontal Therapy), using a high powered phase-contrast microscope may look for pathogens in the scrapings from pockets. The dentist can then assess the presence and extent of infection.

(7) The LINGUAL ASCORBIC ACID TEST by DENTAL DIAGNOSTIC SERVICES, INC., measures the tissue levels of vitamin C which correlates with the health of gums, tooth mobility, pocket depth, jaw bone loss, plaque and calculus accumulation.

(8) Culturing and assay methods may be used to disclose periodontopathogens. These methods are too expensive to be used routinely but may be used in refractory cases to help determine the appropriate antibiotic to be used.

31. QUESTIONS REGARDING DIAGNOSTIC TESTS

Many of the questions below have not been adequately addressed by the makers or proponents of the diagnostic tests. Some tests detect only bacteria which may or may not be pathogenic. Some tests may be capable of detecting the infections that deepen the pocket or erode the supporting bone. Before I can recommend any one of these tests, the questions below need to be answered. Ask your dentist about his opinion.

(1) Does it detect all periodontal infections or periodontopathogens, even at the base of the deepest pockets?

(2) Does it more conveniently and accurately detect infection than traditional clinical and home methods?

(3) Can it detect or predict an upcoming infection?

(4) Can it signal the onset of a disease before the manifestation of symptoms?

(5) Can it detect infection before any damage occurs?

(6) Must all the sites (up to 192) be probed or only symptomatic or deep pockets?

(7) Are the results known during your dental visit?

(8) Is this test available for home-use?

(9) How expensive is it?

32. AFTER YOUR DENTAL VISIT

"Post-prophylaxis periodontal infections" or gum infections due to dental probing, scaling and polishing are common among people suffering from periodontitis. To help prevent these usually minor infections, your dentist should take precaution during your visit. You can help prevent these infections from spreading or developing into an abscess by following the suggestions listed below, immediately after the visit or when you get home.

(1) If no antiseptic mouth rinse was provided for you or if you saw blood during your visit, make an antiseptic solution by adding one teaspoon salt and/or 7 to 14 drops 35% food grade hydrogen peroxide to a one ounce cup of warm water. Swish solution vigorously in your mouth.

(2) If an antibiotic solution was applied in the crevice or pocket and there was some overflow or spillage in the oral cavity, then **gently** brush your teeth and rinse thoroughly with warm water. See section 70(2).

(3) Take vitamin C-NBT for at least a couple of days after your visit especially if you saw blood. See section 84.

(4) If your gums are inflamed from the probing, scaling and polishing, be more gentle when brushing, irrigating and flossing. Try not to irritate them any more. Swash more often.

(5) Be on the alert for infection or abscess formation and deal with them promptly before they do any damage. See PART XI - TREATING GUM INFECTIONS.

PART IV
PERIODONTAL PROCEDURES

33. ROOT SCALING, ROOT PLANING AND CURETTAGE

Root scaling, root planing and curettage do not stop nor reverse the damage due to periodontitis. Some dentists hold the view that pockets cannot be maintained infection-free without them. If or when these procedures fail to stop the pockets from deepening and eroding the bone that supports the teeth your dentist will likely recommend gum surgery to you. Weigh what your dentist says with the outline below.

(1) If you elect any of these procedures, do them at least one month after following THE SMILE METHOD. Your gum health may have improved enough by then that the recovery from these procedures will be shortened.

(2) **Root scaling** (deep or subgingival scaling) is performed to remove calculus from the tooth below the gum line and in the pocket. It is thought that the calculus below the gum line irritates the gum tissue and provides shelter for periodontopathogens. If the calculus accumulates and forms an obstruction similar to a ledge that prevents or makes the insertion of the VITAPICK tip difficult, then ask your dentist to remove it. See "ledge" in diagram near section 66(5).

(3) **Root planing** shaves off or removes part of the tooth surface below the gum line in order to make it smooth.

   (a) To really do a thorough and careful job, root planing requires a lot of time and patience by the dentist. Due to the heavy reliance on tactile sensation, meticulous root planing is technically difficult and dangerous.

   (b) Root planing may make the teeth hypersensitive and more prone to decay.

   (c) There is evidence that a smoother tooth surface creates a difficult environment for bacteria to thrive. Root planing can temporarily reduce gum infections. It may also help the gum tissue partially reattach and thus slightly decrease pocket depth.

(d)   Even if done to perfection this is not a definitive procedure and may have to be repeated.

(4)   **Curettage** is performed with a sharp instrument to scrape away the infected gum tissue inside deep pockets. Curettage especially should be avoided since THE SMILE METHOD will eliminate the gum tissue infection.

(5)   Root scaling, root planing and curettage is initially expensive in time and money. The many follow-up visits often spaced every three months will require even more of these expenditures.

(6)   The potential for infection after any of these procedures are performed is very high.

(a)   Your dentist may use a subgingival applicator or the VITAPICK to apply in your pockets an antiseptic such as hydrogen peroxide and saturated salt solution, or a very well diluted chloramine T. solution. This may sting considerably, so ask your dentist to try (b) instead. See section 74(3).

(b)   After any of these procedures your dentist may deliver an antibiotic solution to the base of the pocket. He will use a subgingival applicator to eject the equivalent of a drop or two of this solution (probably 40 mg tetracycline per ml of water). This may have to be repeated in the following days. You can accomplish the same at home with the VITAPICK. See section 74(4).

(c)   Systemic antibiotics are to be taken only if they cannot be applied at the base of the pocket. See section 68.

(d)   Take mega dose of vitamin C but preferably C-NBT before and after the procedure to help ward off infection. Vitamin C will complement the locally applied and systemic antibiotics that your dentist may prescribe.

(7)   Follow your dentist's advice on what to do immediately after these procedures, then slowly integrate THE SMILE METHOD.

34. GUM SURGERY - PROS AND CONS

The surgical removal of gum tissue to reduce pocket depth to less than 3 mm deep is the prevalent view held by dentists and periodontists on how to treat periodontitis. The deeper the pockets the more likely and the more urgently the surgery will be recommended. This is due to the belief that cutting away the gum tissue makes these areas accessible to the toothbrush and thus can be maintained infection-free. Before deciding for or against surgery, you along with your dentist should assess the risks involved and the possible benefits that may be derived. Listed below are the advantages and disadvantages for this procedure to help you decide.

(1) **Gum surgery does not cure periodontitis.** It does not repair the damage that has taken place. The cutting away of the gum tissue is considered a destructive procedure (it can not be reversed).

(2) **It does initially stop most bleeding.** It may also reduce abscess formation and improve breath odor.

(3) **It is not a definitive procedure.** Many people suffer a relapse hence the surgery may have to be repeated. Often people who elected to have gum surgery once opt for obvious reasons not to have it performed a second time.

(4) **It is dangerous.** All surgery from the so-called simple up to the most intricate kind, involves some degree of danger to one's health.

  (a) Any time there is cutting into tissue and blood flows, there is a chance for infection and physical damage.

  (b) Gum surgery may require up to 30 incisions and even more stitches.

  (c) Danger also arises due to the extensive use of pain killers and systemic antibiotics for up to two weeks after each surgical session.

(5) **It is expensive.** Gum surgery takes money away from your pocket book and time away from your life, due to many (up to twenty) dental visits required. In 1997 dollars it costs $400 to $1500 per quadrant or $1600 to $6000 total for all four quadrants. Do not let the fact that your health insurance covers gum surgery sway you to have it performed.

(6) **It is painful!** With all (as many as forty) oral injections given to block pain, most people do not find the surgery itself painful; however osseous surgery or reshaping by drilling away some of the supporting bone is painful even with pain killing injections. Depending on the extent of the surgery, post operative pain and discomfort may last up to five days.

(7) **It is disfiguring.** Since some of the gum is cut back, more of the root is exposed making your teeth longer, which can make you look older. This may become obvious when you smile. Gum tissue does not regenerate.

(8) **It increases sensitivity.** Surgery requires that the gum is cut back which exposes more of the dentin. This often causes the teeth to become more sensitive to hot or cold drinks and other stimuli. This hypersensitivity may last a few weeks or may go on for many years. See section 96.

(9) **It is not maintenance-free.**

    (a) The daily maintenance routine your dentist or periodontist will prescribe to you after surgery may take more time and often more money than THE SMILE METHOD outlined herein for the avoidance of gum surgery.

    (b) This maintenance routine (as well as THE SMILE METHOD) must be followed daily. It is said that much, if not all, of the improvement to gum health is not due to the surgery but to the added attention that you devote to the care of your gums following the daily maintenance routine.

    (c) The long term effect on your gum health is primarily dependent on the effectiveness of the maintenance program and not the surgery. The daily routine that your dentist recommends may or may not be adequate to prevent further gum infections and deterioration of the underlying supporting bone. THE SMILE METHOD may be slowly implemented after surgery.

35. DENTAL OFFICE ADVICE

What happens when you walk into a dental office is a well choreographed and orchestrated string of events. Most events are for your benefit, but many are for the profit of the dentist. Nothing wrong with profit, unless this motivation harms you by limiting, ignoring or concealing your options.

(1) Various organizations offer courses to dentists on how to increase profit by motivating you to take their advice regarding your periodontal options. They train the dentist to handle all the objections you may have to gum surgery. This script is rehearsed and memorized.

(2) Do not engage your dentist in an argument regarding the merits of his

treatment versus THE SMILE METHOD. You are not there to win an argument.

    (a)   Your dentist may really believe that gum surgery or whatever he recommends is the way to treat periodontitis. He may not like a home-care program that he did not recommend. He may resist helping you implement your preferred mode of treatment.

    (b)   Your dentist may not trust or believe that you can be motivated and properly instructed by a book. Even with this book in hand you may have a hard time convincing him to assist you in the few items necessary to implement THE SMILE METHOD.

(3)   You are at a disadvantage in making major dental decisions, in the dental offices, seated in the dental chair and looking up at your dentist. The presence or fear of pain may complicate your decision making abilities. Tell your dentist you need time to think about decisions involving all major periodontal procedures and tooth extractions.

36. IF YOU ELECT TO HAVE GUM SURGERY

Gum surgery is not performed on an emergency basis. You will have time to improve your gum health with THE SMILE METHOD. If you elect to have surgery consider the following:

(1)   Read up on gum surgery! Ask your dentist for literature or write or call the AMERICAN DENTAL ASSOCIATION and AMERICAN ACADEMY OF PERIODONTOLOGY. The information that you obtain may help you decide if you should use your dentist or use a periodontist. Learn about the various surgical procedures available and what results to expect. See section 23 for addresses and phone numbers.

(2)   Ask family and friends who had gum surgery for recommendations.

(3)   Inform your dentist of the following:

    (a)   Any ailments especially of any heart related ailments you have or had.

    (b)   Any drugs that you may be taking.

    (c)   Any allergies to antibiotics, local anesthesia or other drugs.

    (d)   Women should inform their dentist if pregnant.

(4)   A few days before gum surgery, start taking C-NBT. Do likewise after

surgery. Antibiotics will undoubtedly be prescribed by your dentist to protect you against local and systemic infection. Vitamin C, especially C-NBT promotes healing, improves your immune system, and increases the effectiveness of antibiotics while simultaneously reducing allergic reaction to them.

PART V
ANTISEPTICS

37. WHICH ANTISEPTICS TO USE - OUTLINE

Baking soda, salt solution, hydrogen peroxide and colloidal silver are antiseptics that have a long safety record when used as recommended. The first three are natural, anti-inflammatory and economical. All have been tested extensively and have been shown to be effective against bacteria that promote periodontitis. Liquid antiseptic dentifrices are used because liquids have the properties of capillary attraction and osmosis. Liquids can penetrate the smallest crevice and are easily diffused in the crevicular fluid where many periodontopathogens are found.

(1) **Baking soda** (soda, sodium bicarbonate, bicarbonate of soda) is mostly known under the ARM AND HAMMER label. Use baking soda not baking powder.

    (a) Its high alkalinity (pH 8 to 9) neutralizes harmful acids.

    (b) It is slightly abrasive, when dry and excellent for mechanically removing plaque. It is less abrasive than most commercial dentifrices.

    (c) It loses its abrasive property and acts more like an antiseptic as it turns into a slurry, which then easily dissolves in water or saliva.

    (d) Use a lot of it when manual-brushing.

    (e) When soda is used to make solutions (instead of salt) use about one teaspoon of it per one ounce of water.

    (f) The AMERICAN DENTAL ASSOCIATION COUNCIL OF AMERICAN DENTAL THERAPEUTICS has approved baking soda to be used as a dentifrice.

(2) Use **table salt** (sodium chloride), regular, sea or iodized.

    (a) Salt in solution is not abrasive. Do not brush with salt crystals.

    (b) When making a saturated salt solution for the irrigator, avoid using more salt than the amount that will dissolve in warm water when stirred.

(c) When making all other saturated salt solutions in the one ounce measuring cup, use a little more salt than the amount that totally dissolves. The undissolved salt will settle on the bottom.

(d) Use a half to one teaspoon salt per ounce of water. Use no more than two tablespoons in eight ounces of water.

(3) Use **hydrogen peroxide** preferably the 35% food grade.

(a) It is especially effective against anaerobic bacteria and may be able to detoxify some noxious bacterial by-products.

(b) Add to water to dilute between 0.35% to 1.0% before usage. See section 43, HYDROGEN PEROXIDE - SAFETY WARNING.

(c) Over the long term do not use hydrogen peroxide on a daily basis when brushing or irrigating. On a regular basis you may use it every second or third day. For short periods, it may be used several times per day. It may be added to the salt solution to increase the potency.

(4) Use **colloidal silver** in the VITAPICK applicator only. Apply the equivalent of approximately one or two drops per pocket.

(a) It is effective against many pathogenic bacteria.

(b) Use colloidal silver containing between 5 to 60 p.p.m. (parts per million) silver. The higher concentration is more potent. Colloidal silver made by electrocolloidal process with the smallest particle size is preferred.

(c) Colloidal silver does not sting like salt solution or hydrogen peroxide when applied in an infected pocket. It may however cause a very brief tingle due to the contact of the solution on the infected site in the pocket.

(d) You may use colloidal silver daily. It is safe to use. People drink it for health reasons. You may swish the overflow, but as a precaution do not swallow it.

(e) The FDA is in the process of banning all colloidal silver and mild silver protein products for sale over the counter. Will they succeed?

38. HOW THE ANTISEPTICS ARE USED - OUTLINE

In THE SMILE METHOD, antiseptics are used for brushing, irrigating, flossing and in the applicator.

(1)   Dip a manual-brush or INTERPLAK (and maybe other electric-brushes) in a saturated salt or in a salt and 0.35% to 1.0% hydrogen peroxide solution. For mixing information see section 49(2).

(2)   On a BIOTENE toothbrush saturated with warm water add 1 or 2 drops of 35% hydrogen peroxide. On other manual-brushes saturate with water and add 1 drop of 35% hydrogen peroxide. See section 49(3).

(3)   On a manual-brush saturated with water add 1 drop of 35% hydrogen peroxide then dip in baking soda. See section 49(1).

(4)   In the irrigator use a saturated salt **or** a salt and 0.35% to 1.0% hydrogen peroxide solution. For mixing information see section 57.

(5)   Floss with baking soda. See section 72(4).

(6)   In the VITAPICK use a saturated salt **or** a salt and 0.35% to 1.0% hydrogen peroxide solution. See section 74.

(7)   Use colloidal silver in the VITAPICK applicator only. See section 74(3).

(8)   Apply Tea Tree Oil near infected site. See section 72(3).

(9)   For mouthwash or gargle use a 0.5% to 1.0% hydrogen peroxide solution. See section 92(1).

   (a)   Add 10 drops of 35% hydrogen peroxide to an **one ounce** cup of warm water (to yield a 0.7% solution).

   (b)   Add one teaspoon (5 ml) of 35% hydrogen peroxide to an **eight ounce** cup of warm water (to yield a 0.7% solution).

   (c)   For a more potent solution add salt and stir.

39. HYDROGEN PEROXIDE

In THE SMILE METHOD, hydrogen peroxide is relied on often. Note the following:

(1)   Its chemical designation is H_2O_2. It is composed of two parts hydrogen and two parts oxygen, one more oxygen atom than water. When it comes in contact with plaque it effervesces, freeing the extra oxygen atom and

turning the remainder into water.

(2)   Oxygen can destroy viral, bacterial and fungal pathogens. It detoxifies many bacterial toxins.

(3)   Hydrogen peroxide is effective against many of the periodontopathogens which are thought to be anaerobic, that is they thrive in a low or oxygen free environment. Hydrogen peroxide releases oxygen which is fatal to anaerobic bacteria.

(4)   Your white blood cells produce hydrogen peroxide to kill bacteria. Many of your body cells produce hydrogen peroxide. Bacteria associated with health produce peroxide compounds.

(5)   Highly dilute solution of hydrogen peroxide has been injected and infused intravenously for various ailments apparently without any harm. This is not to say that hydrogen peroxide is harmless but that when properly used it is both safe and effective.

40. 35% AND 3% HYDROGEN PEROXIDE COMPARED

Hydrogen peroxide is available in two forms:

(1)   **35% food grade hydrogen peroxide**.

    (a)   It may be purchased at some health food stores or by mail. I have tried 35% food grade hydrogen peroxide that was sold as such but was diluted to around 17.5%. The company that was selling it claimed that the contents included 35% food grade hydrogen peroxide but not that the contents were actually so. Experience will tell you that it takes more hydrogen peroxide to do the same job.

    (b)   35% food grade hydrogen peroxide has the added advantage of being edible (at least in diluted form). It is included in the FDA (Food and Drug Administration) GRAS (Generally Recognized As Safe) list of food additives. The good thing about the 35% food grade hydrogen peroxide is that it does not have any buffers or stabilizers added.

    (c)   Dilute it to 1.0% or less, by adding it to water. The 35% hydrogen peroxide because it is highly concentrated, when added to warm water will not change the temperature of the solution. See sections 105 and 107.

(2)   **3% U.S.P.** (United States Pharmacopoeia) hydrogen peroxide solution.

    (a)   The 3% hydrogen peroxide can be found in drugstores and super-markets and may be used if the 35% food grade hydrogen peroxide is not available.

    (b)   The added buffers and stabilizers mixed in it for preservation are undesirable for internal use and not intended to be swallowed. Always rinse mouth after using the 3% U.S.P. hydrogen peroxide solution.

    (c)   Dilute it to 1.0% or less by adding it to warm water. This cools the temperature of the solution more than you may like. See section 106.

    (d)   It is safer to handle though it is more expensive and bulkier than the 35% food grade hydrogen peroxide.

41. HOW TO USE HYDROGEN PEROXIDE

Note the following usage instructions:

(1)   The 35% food grade hydrogen peroxide and the 3% U.S.P. hydrogen peroxide must be diluted.

    (a)   Always use a 1.5% or weaker solution. To dilute the 35% hydrogen peroxide to the proper percentage, convert to equivalent drops or parts. See sections 105, 106 and 107, DILUTING 35% and 3% FOOD GRADE HYDROGEN PEROXIDE.

    (b)   Never use over 1.5% hydrogen peroxide solution on your gums. Such a strong solution may cause tingling or burning sensation in your mouth and sloughing of cheek tissue. The raw parts of your gum and lips may turn white temporarily.

    (c)   Keep in mind that in THE SMILE METHOD the 35% and 3% hydrogen peroxide is diluted between 0.35% to 1.0%.

(2)   Daily overuse, and personal sensitivity to hydrogen peroxide even below 1.5% dilution can form ulcers in the mouth which may be visible and painful. It may also cause pain or discomfort when it comes in contact with hypersensitive teeth.

    (a)   Use a more dilute solution, as low as 0.35%.

(b) Decrease usage to every second or third day. If ulceration or irritation persists discontinue using hydrogen peroxide.

(c) If the mucous membrane in your mouth becomes irritated stop adding hydrogen peroxide on your brush and in the liquid dentifrice. If irritation persists also stop irrigating with it.

(d) To increase potency it is best to always add hydrogen peroxide to the salt solution used in the VITAPICK.

(3) If you have chapped lips and the hydrogen peroxide (or salt) seems to aggravate them, apply aloe vera gel, lip balm, petroleum jelly or salve containing glycerin on them. If that fails then try BLISTEX.

42. HANDLING AND DISPENSING OF HYDROGEN PEROXIDE

Proper handling of 35% food grade hydrogen peroxide is important for safety, efficiency and economy.

(1) The 35% hydrogen peroxide has an excellent shelf life. Long term storage should be in a dark, cool location. It is best to store below 68°F but room temperature is fine.

(2) The medium size (pint?) plastic bottle of 35% hydrogen peroxide is used in conjunction with the irrigator.

(3) Get an one or two ounce plastic drop-dispenser bottle, the type that forms drops when held upside down and squeezed. This comes in handy as some hydrogen peroxide solutions are made by counting drops. You can also accomplish accurate dilution with an eye dropper but it is much more troublesome to use.

(4) Get an one ounce clear plastic measuring cup that can also measure fraction of an ounce, tablespoon, teaspoon and milliliter.

(a) As your personal mixing cup to make liquid dentifrice and to dip brush into.

(b) This is used for measuring the hydrogen peroxide and salt to be poured into the irrigator reservoir.

(c) This is used to measure and mix solutions which are drawn into the VITAPICK.

(d)   This may also be used to rinse your mouth with clean water.

43. HYDROGEN PEROXIDE - SAFETY WARNING

Certain precautions should be taken when using and handling hydrogen peroxide. Carefully read the warnings below and the warnings listed on the label and packaging box.

(1)   **CAUTION:** 35% food grade hydrogen peroxide is a strong oxidizer and a very caustic substance if not properly diluted. It should be properly labelled to prevent accidental misuse.

(2)   **CAUTION:** Avoid contact with skin and especially with eyes and mucous membranes. Upon contact 35% hydrogen peroxide will sting and blanch (turns white) the skin temporarily. Flush with water immediately after contact. If there was contact with eyes, call or visit a physician as soon as possible.

(3)   **CAUTION:** Drinking hydrogen peroxide undiluted or insufficiently diluted can do serious harm. If swallowed accidentally drink water to dilute it. Do not cause vomiting. See a physician.

(4)   **CAUTION: KEEP 35% FOOD GRADE HYDROGEN PEROXIDE** (since it is clear like water), **ANTIBIOTICS, ALL DRUGS AND DANGEROUS SUBSTANCES AWAY FROM THE REACH OF CHILDREN.**

(5)   **CAUTION:** Never use a solution stronger than 1.5% hydrogen peroxide on your gums or teeth.

(6)   Use of hydrogen peroxide may promote on rare occasions the overgrowth of the filiform papillae, and if a fungus is involved you may get a black hairy tongue. Ask your dentist for advice.

44. THE SMILE METHOD AND HIGH BLOOD PRESSURE

Both salt and baking soda contain sodium. If consumed, they can cause the blood pressure to rise in some people. If you have high blood pressure or are on a sodium restricted diet, note the following:

(1)   Accidental swallowing of salt and baking soda during brushing, irrigating or when using the VITAPICK, may contribute to your total sodium

intake. Lean over the sink and let these solutions drain out of your mouth.

(2) Inadequate rinsing after using salt or baking soda may leave a small amount of sodium residue which may be swallowed later. Rinse thoroughly several times with water after using these substances.

(3) Epsom salt (magnesium sulfate) does not contribute to high blood pressure and may be substituted for salt. To substitute brushing with baking soda you may use a saturated Epsom salt warm water solution as dentifrice.

(4) Each 10 gm of sodium ascorbate (a form of vitamin C) contains 1,240 mg of sodium. It may be as high as 3 gm in some brands. See sections 86(3) and 87(2).

PART VI
BRUSHING

45. WHY BRUSH

Brushing is part of THE SMILE METHOD daily routine. In the treatment of periodontitis this task is indispensable.

(1) Brushing does a great job cleaning the teeth above the gum line. This is very helpful since what is above the gum line may effect the health below. This is why it is so important to brush all exposed tooth surfaces and tongue and brush/massage the gums.

(2) Much of the benefit derived from brushing is due to the design of the toothbrush and technique used. Mechanical removal of food particles, plaque, debris and stains from teeth is the primary reason to brush. If no dentifrice is available, brush using tap water.

(3) Though helpful, brushing alone is not enough to prevent or eliminate gum infections. Brushing used with the proper antiseptic dentifrice can prevent many and even eliminate some shallow pocket infections.

46. WHEN TO BRUSH

When and how often you brush are as important as the technique and the dentifrice used.

(1) **Manual-brush thoroughly in the morning** after breakfast or before leaving the house. Brush with baking soda most of the time. If you have mastered your brushing technique, a thorough and adequate brushing should take about a minute to perform.

(2) If it is convenient, manual-brush after every meal. A quick warm water brushing and rinsing can be done in less than 15 seconds. This will do a fairly good job at cleaning your teeth, so do not avoid brushing because you feel you do not have the time.

(3) If you cannot brush after meals or snacks that contain refined carbohydrates, especially sugar, swish water vigorously in mouth and rinse several times with water. This will remove some loose plaque but more

important, it will dislodge and eliminate the sugar that is attached to the teeth.

(4) If no water is available then swash. See PART XII.

(5) Brush with an electric-brush once a day preferably **during your bed-time program.** Don't miss this as it is more important than manual-brushing, though not a substitute for it. It only takes about a minute or so to use.

47. HOW TO BRUSH YOUR TEETH

Throughout the years, many methods for brushing teeth have been researched and recommended. All of these methods for brushing are nearly equally good at cleaning the surface of the teeth. The use of an electric-brush and various brands of manual-brushes will make up some of the deficiency in the method or technique that you use to brush. The important thing is to brush.

(1) Ask your dentist or dental hygienist to show you how to brush. They can do a better job showing you than anyone can describing it in writing and can detect and inform you of any bad brushing habits you may have inadvertently acquired. Read the brushing instructions that come with the manual-brushes and especially the electric-brushes.

(2) You may run hot or warm water over the brush just prior to brushing to soften the bristles. The stiffer the bristles the longer you should run hot water over them. Your comfort level should determine the time element and water temperature to use.

(3) Grip brush in a manner you find comfortable and apply dentifrice in one of the following ways:

   (a) Dip manual-brush in baking soda then brush teeth. Repeat dipping and brushing several times. See section 49(1).

   (b) Prepare a salt or salt and hydrogen peroxide warm water solution. Dip manual-brush or electric-brush in liquid dentifrice then brush teeth. Repeat dipping and brushing several times. See section 49(2).

   (c) Add one or two drops of hydrogen peroxide on a brush <u>saturated</u> with water then brush teeth. See section 49(3).

(4) Clench teeth and brush the outside (facial) surfaces of the upper and lower teeth with up and down and circular motion, first clockwise then counter clockwise. The brushing should overlap the gum. This helps clean the gum line and massage the gum. See section 48(3).

(5) Many dentists recommend that you tilt the brush 45° in such a way that the edge of the bristles will clean the gum crevice. If your dentist recommends it or you are happy with the results you achieve by brushing this way, then continue to brush in this manner. The use of some electric-brushes, irrigating and flossing may not necessitate 45° brushing.

(6) **CAUTION:** The idea is to clean your teeth and gum line, not to wear down your teeth or irritate your gum.

   (a) Brush the teeth gently but vigorously enough to remove debris and plaque. Brushing with very heavy pressure can slowly erode the enamel. Inspect your teeth in the mirror to see if your brushing has "gouged" any teeth or formed a "track" (notch or groove) across one or several teeth. If you are not sure what to look for then ask your dentist to check.

   (b) The use of stiff or hard brushes or inadequately softened with hot water coupled with applying too much pressure can make the gum line slowly recede. Never brush so hard that you feel discomfort, pain or that you irritate your gums.

   (c) If the gums are sore or tender, then brush very lightly. You may use the BIOTENE supersoft toothbrush or avoid brushing for a day or two.

   (d) Depending on the severity of your periodontitis take five to twenty days to slowly and gently integrate the use of the electric-brush into your daily routine. Read the manufacturer's recommendations.

(7) Brush the inside (lingual) of the upper and then lower teeth with short back and forth strokes. See TOOTH DESIGNATIONS in section 25.

(8) Brush across missing teeth and on the accessible sides of all four molars and pay special attention under the bridgework.

(9) Finally, brush the chewing surfaces of all four sets of your back teeth with short back-and-forth strokes.

(10) Repeat the brushing sequence 3(a) or 3(b), 4, 7, 8 and 9 (which are noted in bold) two or three times.

(11) If you are using a liquid dentifrice take whatever is left over in the measuring cup and vigorously swish it in mouth forcing it through the gaps between the teeth on the left side, right side and finally the front.

(12) Expectorate excess. Rinse mouth thoroughly with water unless you plan to irrigate or floss.

48. ADDITIONAL MOUTH CLEANING ADVICE

Besides brushing your teeth, there are a few more tasks which will help you maintain healthy gums.

(1)   It is advisable to clean the top surface of your tongue.

    (a)   You may gently scrape it with a spoon in a forward motion from the back towards the tip.

    (b)   You may find that using a brush is more effective at removing debris. Try using the RADIUS D.D.S. toothbrush which has soft bristles and a large surface area. Use a gentle circular then forward motion on the upper surface of the tongue, where debris tends to collect.

    (c)   Do not use an abrasive dentifrice (baking soda slurry is OK.) when brushing your gums or tongue.

    (d)   Never use an electric-brush to clean the top surface of your tongue. Never brush the bottom side of your tongue. Though some dentists may recommend to also manual-brush the inside of your cheeks, I for the most part do not agree with this practice.

(2)   Interdental brushes are tiny brushes that can fit in small spaces.

    (a)   Furcation involvement is the opening created under the fork of multi-rooted teeth (molars and bicuspids) as the result of severe bone loss and gum recession. Dip the interdental brush in liquid dentifrice or baking soda and carefully brush in the furcation. Ask your dentist for advice. See diagram in section 3.

    (b)   If it fits, also brush between troublesome widely spaced teeth using an in and out motion.

    (c)   Interdental brushes are made by BUTLER, DENTEC and other companies and may be purchased at most drugstores.

(3)   You should brush/massage your gums with your manual-brush (or electric-brush if recommended by the manufacturer). Use the same motion that you use to brush your teeth. Massage vigorously but not to the point of irritating your gums. It is best to include this in your bedtime program.

(4) Daily (if you find it necessary or helpful) or once every week or two at maximum, massage your gums with your index finger or thumb. You may want to massage your gums by gripping them with your thumb and index finger.

   (a) This will help circulation.

   (b) This will help you locate abnormalities on your gums that may be diagnosed as an infection.

   (c) Massage your gums prior to using the VITAPICK.

(5) The use of gum stimulators has not been shown to prevent or treat gum infections. I don't recommend using them, but if your dentist does and you find them helpful and you have the time and patience then use them.

49. DENTIFRICES

Below is a list of the ways to mix and use baking soda, salt and 35% food grade hydrogen peroxide to be used as a dentifrice.

(1) Get **baking soda** in the 8 or 16 ounce box which is best suited for this.

   (a) Dip moist brush into the box or pour the soda into palm of hand if you are sharing the contents with someone else. Use a lot of soda; it's economical.

   (b) Occasionally for more effectiveness, prior to dipping the manual-brush into the soda, you may add one drop of 35% hydrogen peroxide directly on the bristles saturated with water. Never add 35% hydrogen peroxide to dry bristles.

   (c) Though some people may not like the taste of baking soda (or salt), most people get used to it in a couple of weeks and often later end up preferring it over flavored commercial dentifrices.

(2) Here is how to make and use the **liquid dentifrice**:

   (a) Add a teaspoon or so of salt to a clean one ounce clear plastic measuring cup. Fill with warm tap water.

   (b) To increase potency add seven (as few as 5 but no more than 14) drops of 35% food grade hydrogen peroxide. Add the hydrogen peroxide to the salt solution every second or third day. For prevention of infection, use a lower percentage. To eliminate infection, you may use a higher percentage. See section 41.

(c) Dip manual-brush or the electric-brush (read manufacturer's instructions to see if this is okay) into solution, then brush teeth. Dip brush to soak up more of the solution then brush again.

(d) When you finish brushing, take the remainder of the solution and swish it in your mouth. Expectorate excess.

(e) The formula used to make the liquid dentifrice may also be used in the VITAPICK, as a mouthwash or gargle.

(3) Occasionally or when in a hurry try this: Fully saturate manual-brush with warm water and add one drop of 35% hydrogen peroxide. Brush teeth and expectorate excess but you need not rinse mouth with water. This is a good time to swash.

50. COMMERCIAL DENTIFRICES

Many toothpaste commercials make promises but fall short on delivery. Though I recommend baking soda, salt and hydrogen peroxide, you may want to try the following products:

(1) There are many "natural" and fluoride-free products available to put on your brush. Some of these products may be as effective as baking soda, salt or hydrogen peroxide (or maybe even more effective?). A few may even claim to cure periodontitis (they do not). Some are flavored and you may like using them better than baking soda, salt solution or hydrogen peroxide.

(2) Toothpastes that contain baking soda are not as effective as using the ingredient full strength. Some toothpastes include hydrogen peroxide to increase effectiveness.

(3) MERFLUAN tooth powder comes in three flavors. Mint, cinnamon and mint or anise. It does not contain fluoride. It's a product worth trying.

(4) PEELU tooth powder has good whitening and antiseptic qualities. Try it!

(5) Many toothpastes and the drinking water in many cities contain fluoride.

(a) The anti-plaque commercial slogans promoting fluoride mean little, since the plaque below the gum line is not effected by it.

(b) Low levels of fluoride are not effective against periodontopathogens and useless in treating periodontitis.

(c) **CAUTION:** The cumulative effects of daily consumption even of very low levels of fluoride may be carcinogenic. There is much controversy in this area. More research is required.

51. MANUAL - BRUSHES

The characteristics or specifications of a toothbrush determine to a great degree its effectiveness. Following are some suggestions for picking a manual-brush.

(1) Choose a toothbrush with a straight handle unless of course you find another shape more comfortable to use.

(2) Get a brush of the proper size with three or four rows of tufts that you find easy to use. Usually these brushes are labelled "adult".

(3) Get a brush that has the following bristles characteristics:

(a) The bristles should be made of nylon. If you have acrylic veneers ask your dentist if nylon bristles will wear them down faster.

(b) The brush should have bristles that flex and follow the contour of the gum and teeth. This helps clean the teeth above and partially below the gum line without damaging the gum crevice. Brushes with nylon bristles .007" or less diameter are recommended. These brushes are designated as soft or extra soft, though there are no established standards for labelling.

(c) Preferably get brushes with the rounded and polished tip bristles which are kinder to the gums.

(4) Brushes with harder bristles (labelled medium or hard) do not follow the contours as well and may damage the teeth and gum tissue.

(5) Generally avoid the natural bristle brushes as they are more expensive, not as durable, have inconsistent quality and are usually very stiff.

52. MANUAL-BRUSHES - PURCHASING

There are many manual-brushes available. Get three or four soft or extra soft toothbrushes and alternate usage. Use various brands and designs as variety increases the effectiveness of brushing. Every year new models are offered.

Experiment with soft and extra soft. I have tested and researched many brushes. Below is a list with comments of some of them.

(1) I highly recommend the BIOTENE supersoft toothbrush for sensitive or irritated gums. This toothbrush is so soft, that it will be difficult to hurt your gums with it. You may therefore brush teeth and gums longer and with a little more pressure.

    (a) Due to the very fine bristles it is not as durable as other brushes. The bristles maintain their form longer if you avoid using it with baking soda.

    (b) It is best to saturate brush with water and add one or two drops of 35% hydrogen peroxide.

    (c) Replace at first sign of bristle curl or when the bristles flare or lose their shape.

(2) Try the BUTLER (John O. Butler Co.) G.U.M. ultra soft toothbrush. Its unique rounded brush shape may clean areas missed by other toothbrushes.

(3) Try the SENSODYNE GENTLE which is a superb extra soft brush. COLGATE also makes an excellent extra soft brush.

(4) Try the ORAL-B which is an all around good soft brush.

(5) Try the RADIUS D-D-S toothbrush which has a soft and large bristle area. This is a big brush for big mouths. It is great for cleaning your teeth flat or at 45° and the top of your tongue. Choose right or left hand model.

(6) Try the DENTRUST which brushes all 3 tooth surfaces at the same time.

(7) For those times when you are away from home and you need to brush, try the BUTLER or similar travel toothbrush. Consider using a disposable brush.

53. ELECTRIC-BRUSH - PURCHASING

Technology has come a long way with the new rechargeable battery operated tooth brush cleaning devices. They are safe and easy to use and may make up for any error in your manual-brushing technique. To a greater or lesser degree all of them kill bacteria in shallow pockets. None however kill bacteria in deep pockets. Prices in 1997 dollars for these electric-brushes vary from between $30 to $150. Unfortunately I have not tried most of these electric-brushes to give a first hand opinion. One through six use mechenical action to dislodge plaque.

(1) The INTERPLAK is truly a well designed toothbrush. This was the brush that sparked the revolution in new designs.

(2) The PLAK TRAC has two counter-rotational heads rather than counter-rotational tufts of the INTERPLAK. Its lower price (almost half of the cost of the INTERPLAK) makes it attractive.

(3) The ORALGIENE (sold by mail) and EPIDENT (sold by dentists) are identical and seem well designed. They brush all six surfaces of the upper and lower teeth at the same time. What a great concept! This could mean fast, error-free brushing.

(4) The BRAUN ORAL-B PLAQUE REMOVER with a larger round rotating brush head seems promising.

(5) The ROTA-DENT (sold only by dentists) and the PROCLEAN2000 are well designed, compact and lightweight electric tooth cleaners. The soft very fine bristles are too tightly bunched but the variety of interchangeable heads adds to its effectiveness. The brush head is small and rotates in one direction which makes it difficult and time consuming to use.

(6) The PROPHY II by SCHERER LABORATORIES (sold only by dentists) utilizes a rubber-like cup with bi-directional rotation. It may be good for polishing teeth but I do not recommend it to be used in the treatment of periodontitis.

(7) The SONICARE by OPTIVA, the SENSONIC by TELEDYNE WATER PIK and the SONIPLAK by AMERICAN DENTRONICS are high frequency sonic brushes. They may be worth trying.

(8) The HYG ION toothbrush by DYNA-DENTAL SYSTEMS uses opposite polarity to dislodge the bacteria clinging to the teeth.

(9) The ULTRASONEX is in a class by itself in that they claim that the ultrasonic waves it generates reach and disorganize the bacterial plaque in deep pockets.

(10) Read the usage and operating instructions that accompanies the electric-brush. Before dipping the brush head in salt solution, read the instructions to verify that it is okay.

(11) **CAUTION:** Electric-brushes that mimic human brushing motion by reciprocating action may be dangerous to use. The oscillating electric-brush may not be as dangerous to use but is less effective at cleaning your teeth and may actually "sweep" the plaque into the gum crevice.

(12) Check consumer periodicals for the latest recommendations on brushes and other dental health products.

54. CARE AND STORAGE OF BRUSHES

Below are some suggestions about how to take care of your manual-brushes. Much also applies to electric-brushes. I advise you to read the manufacturer's manual for their recommendations.

(1) Replace brushes when frayed, splayed or when they begin to flare. Get new brushes yearly (if not sooner).

(2) It is best to let all brushes air dry completely, before reusing them. Drying may take 6 to 24 hours. If you use a soft natural fiber brush, let it air dry for at least 24 hours between usage. This helps to sanitize the bristles.

(3) If you store your manual-brushes in a glass or jar (with handle down), pour in it one ounce of water with 10 drops 35% hydrogen peroxide. This will keep the glass and brush handle tips sanitized.

(4) Toothbrush sanitizers are not necessary due to the air drying. The brush is used with antiseptics or dipped in liquid antiseptic dentifrice before brushing which sanitizes it.

PART VII
IRRIGATING

55. DENTAL IRRIGATORS

Dental irrigators are electric powered devices which pressurize and eject water or solutions in a pulsating stream to the teeth. Irrigating the teeth and gums is one of the tasks of THE SMILE METHOD daily routine.

(1) Its function is to remove food particles and loose plaque from between the teeth and gum crevice. It also delivers the antiseptic solutions into the crevice all around each tooth.

(2) It is effective in areas where brushing and flossing are not. Irrigating has a different function than brushing and flossing and is not a substitute for either one of them.

56. WHEN AND HOW TO IRRIGATE

Proper usage of the irrigator is essential to avoid damaging the gums and ensure effectiveness.

(1) How often you should irrigate, depends on your gum health.

    (a) For preventive purposes, you should irrigate once daily preferably after your last snack or meal as part of your bedtime program.

    (b) Irrigate less frequently, if you find that you still maintain gum health.

    (c) On some days, if for some reason you cannot perform all your tasks then omit irrigating.

    (d) To help eliminate infections in the crevice or shallow pockets, you may carefully irrigate up to two or three times per day.

(2) When first starting to use the irrigator, set the pressure setting on low and slowly and daily increase it until you find the level that is comfortable and effective for you.

    (a) If you are feeling discomfort or pain, it may be that the setting is too high.

(b) It is better to err on the side of safety by setting it too low rather than risk injury by setting it too high.

(c) Once you find the proper setting, leave it there.

(3) The standard tips (which I call "V" tips) that attach to the WATER PIK and most irrigators, concentrate the water stream into a small area. This may be harmful if the pressure setting is set high and the flow is improperly directed. To partially overcome these shortcomings, I developed the U-TIP, a modified irrigation tip that attaches to the WATER PIK. This produces a "blunt" or "broad" stream.

(a) The U-TIP allows you to turn up the setting on the irrigator increasing the flow rate and cleaning efficiency without increasing the chance of infection or damage to your gums.

(b) The increased flow rate shortens the time it takes to irrigate.

(c) I recommend that you try the U-TIP and compare it with the "V" tip.

(4) Some dentists may recommend directing the flow into the gum crevice or pocket. Some say to angle it at 45° at the gum line. I strongly recommend against both of these methods as they may damage the gum or drive debris or plaque further into the gum crevice or even worst into the deep pocket. This can spread or worsen the pocket infection.

(a) The irrigation flow should be directed nearly perpendicular or at around 90° to the tooth surface along the gum line. The stream should be directed to the tooth.

(b) Directing the flow, to the gum or other part of the mouth may cause damage.

(c) It is very easy to get the angle wrong, so to verify that you are irrigating at 90°, occasionally look in the mirror.

(5) Direct the flow to the tooth surface at the gum line and briefly pause between the teeth. Follow the natural contours of the gum line from the outside (facial) upper teeth to the inside (lingual) upper then to the outside lower teeth and finally the inside lower. Repeat this cycle two or three times.

(6) Let the water drain out of your mouth into the sink. Check it for signs of blood. When done, take the leftover solution in the reservoir and vigorously swish in mouth. Expectorate excess.

(7) If you plan to floss, do it while some antiseptic solution still remains in the mouth. If you do not plan to floss, then rinse mouth thoroughly with warm water.

(8) Read the manufacturer's recommendation on how to irrigate. Ask your dentist or dental hygienist to show you how.

(9) **CAUTION:** If your gum health does not improve, your gum infections become more frequent or an abscess is formed and you suspect that irrigating is the cause, you may reduce or stop using the irrigator. You may be improperly doing the following :

    (a) Unintentionally directing the flow into the gum crevice. It is better to direct the stream across the crevice. Be extra careful not to direct the stream into deep pockets.

    (b) Using too high a pressure setting.

    (c) Using too high a concentration of hydrogen peroxide

57. SOLUTIONS TO USE IN THE IRRIGATOR

As part of THE SMILE METHOD, **antiseptic solutions should always be used in the irrigator.** Note the following:

(1) Add warm water to the irrigator reservoir. Using the measuring cup, teaspoon or tablespoon, measure and pour **salt** into it and stir to dissolve it. Baking soda or Epsom salt may be used instead. Use just enough or slightly less ingredients than the amount that will completely dissolve in water.

(2) Using a measuring cup or a calibrated teaspoon, measure and add 35% food grade **hydrogen peroxide** enough to yield a 0.35% to 1.0% hydrogen peroxide solution. Adding hydrogen peroxide makes the solution more potent.

    (a) To help **prevent** gum infections, you may use hydrogen peroxide every second or third day.

    (b) To help **eliminate** infections, you may irrigate with a higher percentage solution.

    (c) Use a 1.0% solution if it does not irritate your gums. Use a lower percentage if it is irritating or if your teeth are hypersensitive to it.

(3) Use the following mixing formula to make a saturated salt solution or a

salt and 0.35% to 1.0% hydrogen peroxide solution. It usually takes about a 10 ounce solution to properly irrigate your gums and teeth. If using 20 or 30 ounces works better for you then use that amount.

(a) Add **10 ounces** of warm water to the reservoir, then pour approximately 30 ml salt. Thereafter add 3 ml to 9 ml 35% hydrogen peroxide and stir.

(b) Add **20 ounces** of warm water to the reservoir then pour approximately 60 ml salt. Thereafter add 6 ml to 18 ml 35% hydrogen peroxide and stir.

(c) Add **30 ounces** of warm water to the reservoir then pour approximately 90 ml salt. Thereafter add 9 ml to 27 ml 35% hydrogen peroxide and stir.

(4) On AQUA FLOSS battery operated irrigator add 8 to 20 drops of 35% hydrogen peroxide to the one ounce measuring cup of warm water. Pour this solution into irrigator. Pour warm water in irrigator and fill to capacity.

58. DENTAL IRRIGATOR - PURCHASING

There are several irrigators presently available. I have personally tested and approve the first two.

(1) The WATER PIK manufactured by TELEDYNE is by far the most popular. It is available in family and individual configurations. It may be bought at many drugstores and discount centers. Some models can handle salt solutions and this is stated as such in the sales literature, on the box or in the instructions. It is reasonably priced.

(2) The SUNBEAN irrigator can be found at some drugstores and discount centers. It is well designed and can handle salt solutions. It is priced near the WATER PIK.

(3) The BRAUN irrigator can be found at some drugstores and discount centers. Verify that the model you are considering can be used with salt solution.

(4) AQUA FLOSS is a battery operated irrigator. It is available at some drugstores or discount centers. It has a small capacity (1.7 ounces) and it is not designed to handle salt solutions. Besides its shortcomings it can be useful to the traveller.

(5)   DR. WOOG PERIOSYSTEM is an irrigator plus electric tooth-brush (oscillating action brush) combined. It is very expensive and sold only through the mail.

(6)   HYDRO FLOSS distributed by OXYFRESH (sold by local distributors) has a built-in permanent magnet which produces a magnetic flux field. The manufacturer claims this partially ionizes the water so that it reduces the formation of plaque and calculus. It will handle salt solutions. It costs roughly three times more than a WATER PIK.

(7)   The life of some of these irrigators can be extended, if you briefly run fresh water through them to flush out the salt residue. The base units may be wall mounted to save on shelf space. Read manufacturer's operating and maintenance instructions for recommendations.

(8)   I do not recommend that you use water pressure operated irrigators that attach to your faucet or shower head. You cannot add antiseptic solutions to these types of irrigators.

PART VIII
FLOSSING

59. FLOSSING

The evidence that flossing is helpful in the treatment of periodontitis is over-whelming. Flossing is one of the tasks of THE SMILE METHOD daily routine.

(1) Flossing breaks up plaque thus preventing it from colonizing.

(2) Flossing mechanically loosens and removes some of the sticky plaque which is inaccessible to the bristles of a toothbrush. It cleans between the teeth and up to 4 mm below the gum line, in the crevice but not in the pockets.

(3) Flossing cannot (neither can brushing and irrigating) dislodge calculus.

(4) If you have not flossed before, your gums may hurt or bleed for five or more days at very tender sites that may or may not be infected. If bleeding persists, at some sites, it may be due to infection. See section 72, TREATING SHALLOW POCKET INFECTIONS.

60. FLOSS

Floss is untwisted or slightly twisted thread composed of hundreds of tiny nylon strands which is used to clean between the teeth.

(1) I recommend that you use thin floss because it is easier to use and can reach deeper into the gum crevice. If you really like thick floss go right ahead and use it.

    (a) Thin, fine or extra fine floss by BUTLER is of high quality and probably the thinnest best floss made.

    (b) PATHMARK, JOHNSON & JOHNSON and GENOVESE also produce a high quality thin floss.

    (c) If shredding is a problem, try GLIDE floss. It easily slips between even the tightest gap. Waxed floss does not shred as easily as unwaxed. Experiment with other brands and your flossing technique.

    (d)   If you really like tape or ribbon then use them, but note that they are all waxed. GENOVESE dental tape is the thinnest available.

(2)   Floss is available waxed or unwaxed.

    (a)   I recommend unwaxed because it has a capacity to absorb. Unwaxed and untwisted floss fans out, thus increasing surface area as it rounds the tooth. To see the fanning effect, floss the edge of a table.

    (b)   If you really like waxed then use it, but note that it may leave an unwanted wax residue.

(3)   Tea Tree Oil impregnated floss by DESERT ESSENCE, astringent floss by BERGAFLUOR and fluoridated floss may be more effective than plain floss in preventing infection in the gum crevice. Fluoridated floss releases such a small amount of fluoride, that it seems unlikely to cause any harm.

(4)   On my wish list is that someone develop and produce a floss that will change colors to disclose the presence of periodontopathogens, occult (hidden) blood or white blood cells, all of which reflect the health of the gums. Better yet, a type of floss may be invented that will attract and remove periodontopathogens or make the gum crevice impervious to infection.

61. WHEN AND WHERE TO FLOSS

Flossing to some people is a difficult and undesirable chore. For this reason I have tried to find alternatives, but unfortunately there just are not any. By following the instructions below, you will become more skilful at it and then you may find it more pleasant.

(1)   Floss once or twice a day. Do not exceed two days between flossing. Experiment! Keep in mind that the detrimental effects of not flossing take a while to become evident. Let the health of your gums determine how often you floss.

(2)   The best time to floss is after your last meal or snack of the day, or as part of your bedtime program.

(3)   Floss in front of a mirror at least until you become proficient at it or during a dental crisis so you can clearly observe the details and consequence of your actions. You may use the lip and cheek retractor if you find it helpful.

(4)   As you become skilled at flossing, it will take much less time to accomplish. Do it when watching TV or listening to music. This way you are doing at least one thing you enjoy.

62. HOW TO FLOSS

Flossing is not the easiest task to learn. Through patience and practice, I am confident that you can master it.

(1)   Follow this procedure:

   (a)   Remove about 30" (80 cm) of floss. It may take more or less for you. Experiment!

   (b)   Wind most of it around the base of the finger nail or the tip of the left middle finger (left handers may reverse the handedness) and about 6" (or 16 cm) around the tip of the right middle finger.

   (c)   Use the index finger instead of the middle finger if it is more convenient for you.

   (d)   Leave about 3" to 6" (8 cm to 16 cm) of floss unwound between the fingers.

   (e)   The right hand is used to take up or "reel up" the soiled floss.

(2)   Use the thumb(s) or index finger(s) to guide the floss between the teeth. Keep the floss taut. Experiment!

(3)   **CAUTION:** Never snap the floss into your gums. This can damage the very delicate gum tissue. Where the space between the teeth is very tight, cautiously (guarding against snapping) "work" the floss in. Use a firm sawing action rather than inward brute force. If you are really having a hard time working it between the teeth then try using lightly or fully waxed floss.

(4)   Wrap the floss around the side of tooth so that it resembles a "U". This enhances effectiveness by increasing the sweep area.

(5)   **Keep the floss under tension against the side of each tooth.** Use a firm up-and-down motion (about five or six times) coupled with a gentle sawing action and scrape each tooth. Floss above and below the gum line. The up-and-down motion seems to be more effective at disrupting the plaque but add the sawing action to help remove it.

(6)   **CAUTION:** Do Not "dig" or cut into the gum crevice with the floss. The pressure should be against the tooth not the crevice or gum tissue.

(7) Floss each side of both adjacent teeth at every tooth spacing and the far side of your four back teeth. Start anywhere on the upper teeth and finish wherever you please on the lowers. Be systematic and floss all the teeth. It is not necessary that your teeth make a "squeaky clean" sound to indicate cleanliness.

(8) If your gum bleeds or feels "raw" when flossing you may add a baking soda and maneuver it into the crevice. See section 72(4).

(9) The used up floss may harbor periodontopathogens, especially from infected sites.

   (a) Make sure you use fresh floss on each tooth to avoid cross contamination. Store the soiled floss by taking it up (or "reeling it up") on the right middle finger.

   (b) Avoid touching the soiled floss on lips, as this may cause an infection at the point of contact.

   (c) If you have a cold sore on lip which is further irritated by flossing use the lip and cheek retractor. This will protect the sore from the floss.

(10) Rinse **thoroughly** with warm water after flossing. Look in the mirror and smile!

(11) If the floss snags or shreds, it may be due to inlays or caps with overhangs and ledges, fillings or calculus build-up. If change of floss or technique has not helped then discuss this problem with your dentist. See diagram in section 66(5).

(12) The floss can break and leave a potion jammed tightly between your teeth. Do not attempt to force the jammed floss towards the gum in order to remove it. To avoid injury feed a floss threader below the jammed floss and push it out away from the gum. See section 63(5a).

(13) Ask your dentist or dental hygienist to show you how to floss or for more details read the instructions on the floss package.

63. FLOSSING AIDS

Many devices now available promise to make flossing easier or at least more effective. The best way to floss is the old fashioned tried and true method described earlier. If you are having difficulties properly flossing using that method, then try one of the following:

(1)   BUTLER makes the FLOSSMATE, an inexpensive "Y" shaped plastic dental floss handle. PREVENTIVE DENTISTRY PRODUCTS INC. produces the EZ DENTAL FLOSSER PLUS. If you try to use fresh floss on each site as you should, they become cumbersome to use. The other problem is that the floss is always taut and unyielding thus preventing the floss from wrapping like a "U" partially around the tooth.

(2)   There are several electric flossers now available that claim to be more effective and easier to use. Use flossers that automatically take-up the soiled floss while reeling out the fresh floss. This is to avoid inserting the soiled floss in the crevice. I have not researched the safety and effectiveness of any of these products.

(3)   DR. FLOSSER by FLOSSRITE CORP. is a floss holder with automatic tension, dispensing and soiled floss take-up. It seems like a good design but unfortunately I have not researched the safety and effectiveness of this product.

(4)   Several companies make multi-purpose disposable floss holders, toothpick or gum stimulator combinations.

    (a)   The floss in these products is fixed and taut. This does not allow the floss to partially wrap around the tooth in the form of a "U".

    (b)   I do not recommend these because of possible site cross-contamination and because soiled floss loses its absorptive ability

    (c)   If you find them useful and if used only once and discarded, then use them. They are great if you are on the move.

(5)   To floss under a bridge, between connected caps and splinted teeth, you need a floss threader.

    (a)   Try the BUTLER EEZ-THRU floss threader or other similar product. Though it is more troublesome to floss these teeth, you should nevertheless floss them as often as the others.

    (b)   On my wish list is that someone produce a "bridge-floss" to speed up feeding the floss under the bridgework. This will be made of thin floss in the standard container but every 14" there will be a 2" tinted semi-rigid segment that will be used to feed under the bridge.

PART IX
DEEP POCKETS

64. DEEP POCKET DELIVERY SYSTEMS

In the treatment of periodontitis there has always been a problem in preventing and eliminating the damaging deep pocket infections. None of the routine tasks such as brushing, flossing, irrigating and swashing reach the base (apex or the deepest part of a pocket) let alone eliminate deep pocket infections. Neither does scaling. These procedures can only reach the gum crevice or shallow pockets. There are several ways now available that deliver antiseptic and antibiotic solutions to kill the bacteria at these difficult to reach sites.

(1)   My research has led to the development of the VITAPICK. This practical home-use, deep pocket applicator is inexpensive, small, light, easy to use. It can produce the proper pressure to deliver solutions to the base of the deepest pocket.

    (a)   The VITAPICK is used to deliver or apply a minute amount of **antiseptic** or **antibiotic** solution. These solutions are delivered through a very thin tip (cannula, blunt needle) to the base of deep pockets.

    (b)   **THE VITAPICK APPLICATOR IS THE BEST WAY TO ELIMINATE DEEP POCKET INFECTIONS.** Without it you cannot kill the bacteria that cause infections and periodontal abscesses in deep pockets. See section 74(3) and (4).

    (c)   **THE VITAPICK USED PERIODICALLY IS THE SINGLE MOST IMPORTANT WAY TO PREVENT DEEP POCKET INFECTIONS FROM RECURRING.** See section 74(3).

    (d)   The VITAPICK can be obtained locally or direct. See section 19(1).

(2)   Home irrigators like the WATER PIK with the "standard tip" (or "V" tip) should not be used to try to force antiseptic solutions to the base of deep pockets. To try to reach the base requires such great pressure that it will damage the delicate gum tissue. This can also force the bacteria further in the pocket spreading or worsening the infection.

(3) The "sulcus tips" that some manufacturers of irrigators recommend to use to irrigate deep pockets are too big to enter the pocket let alone reach the base.

(4) The standard tip with cannula attached that fit the WATER PIK or other irrigators are impractical for self-treatment.

    (a) The pulsating stream vibrates the connected hose and tip making it difficult to insert into the pocket.

    (b) The tip is usually connected to a spring loaded spiral hose which restricts maneuverability.

    (c) Often the tip is too big for safe entry into the pocket.

    (d) The reservoir's large capacity makes it impractical to dispense a minute dose of antiseptic and antibiotic.

(5) The difficult procedure of packing baking soda (which may be mixed with hydrogen peroxide) into a pocket with a toothpick has been tried with limited success. Vitamin C at high dosage levels tightens the gums around the teeth which makes this procedure more difficult. It is nevertheless worth trying on shallow pockets.

(6) TELEDYNE produces the PERIOPIK for the dental profession. It can be used to irrigate the crevice or apply a small mount of antiseptics or antibiotic solution to the base of deep pockets.

(7) A plastic squeeze bottle with cannula available from some dentists is very difficult to use. It cannot produce adequate pressure to deliver solutions to the base of deep pockets.

(8) The VITAPICK deep pocket applicator opens up many possibilities for research and development of solutions that will eliminate or prevent recurrence of deep pocket infections more quickly and for a longer duration than salt solution, hydrogen peroxide and colloidal silver. All solutions considered must be known to be safe over many years of usage.

    (a) Diluted BETADINE and HIBICLENS are two solutions that warrant further study. Others: mild silver protein, grapefruit seed extract, calendula tincture and iodine. Herb extracts and essential oils should also be considered. DMSO may be considered as a carrier. Unfortunately it (and Tea Tree Oil) shortens the life of the rubber plunger used in the VITAPICK.

(b)   On my wish list is that someone develop and produce an antiseptic that is as effective as antibiotics, but without the potential risks. An antibiotic that will be safe to use regularly to prevent or eliminate gum infections, may also be considered for research.

(c)   Diagnosis of a gum infection is the weakest link in the treatment of periodontitis. So that the patient is not guessing about their gum health, I also add to my wish list that the new solutions provide a painless way to disclose the presence of infection.

65. LOCATING DEEP POCKETS

Deep pockets are those that are more than 4 mm to 12 mm (1/2") or so deep. If you are a candidate for gum surgery or root planing then you have deep pockets. You must know where your deep pockets are located for prevention and treatment of infections.

(1)   When you are at your dentist's office, note the following:

(a)   Ask your dentist to point out the location of all your deep pockets while the periodontal probe is inserted. See section 28(2).

(b)   Ask him to mark all the pocket depths on a chart. Get a copy of the chart for your use and put a red dot where pockets **over** 4 mm deep are located.

(c)   To gain experience and learn how it feels to insert the applicator, ask your dentist to let you insert the periodontal probe in your pockets. See diagrams near sections 20(4) and 66(5).

(2)   Put your dental chart in a plastic sleeve and hang it in your washroom near or on a mirror for fast, easy reference.

(3)   Deep pockets are more likely to be found between the teeth. Molars generally have deeper pockets than front teeth. Some teeth may have more than one deep pocket. To locate shallow and deep pockets on your own with the applicator do the following:

(a)   Fill the VITAPICK with a salt and hydrogen peroxide solution. See section 74(3).

(b)   **Keep the tip in contact with the tooth.** This will help guide you into the gum crevice and help avoid irritating or piercing the gum. See diagram near section 66(5).

(c)   Carefully insert the tip in the crevice. Gently "walk" and wiggle the tip in the gum crevice around each tooth.

(d) While probing, simultaneously slowly release some antiseptic solution. This makes insertion easier and protects against infection.

(e) "Feel" your way around each tooth and into the pocket.

(4) Deep pockets are more likely to be symptomatic, get infected and form an abscess.

66. HOW TO USE THE VITAPICK

Once you use the VITAPICK applicator several times and it becomes routine, you will find that this procedure is not painful. Some pockets are easily accessible while others may require some experimentation to insert the tip.

(1) Prepare the appropriate antiseptic or antibiotic solution. See sections 74(3) and 74(4).

(a) The VITAPICK can be filled to capacity. It is usually better however to employ the **drop technique** in which you draw in only one or two drops. Using the VITAPICK or an eye dropper apply many drops of the solution on a clean surface like a dish and draw in one or two drops at a time. The **fill to capacity technique** is faster to use but does not allow you control of dispensing minute doses. The drop technique allows you full control when it is necessary to apply additional pressure to deliver the minute dose to the base of the pocket. The low dose reduces stinging and is more economical to use.

(b) To fill applicators, submerge tip and draw in the solution. Keep the tip submerged to avoid drawing air bubbles. If air bubbles are formed, invert the applicator. Tap to float the air bubbles then push plunger to eject them. **CAUTION: Be extra careful not to get any solution in your eyes.**

(c) To avoid clogging the tip, fill from near the surface of the solution, not from the bottom where the undissolved salt or antibiotic may have settled.

(d) **CAUTION:** If the tip gets clogged, do not attempt to force the solution through. This could eject the tip like a projectile and inflict bodily injury. Clogged tips usually cannot be salvaged.

(2) I highly recommend you use a lip and cheek retractor. The results are not quite as good but you make your teeth and gums more visible and accessible by extending your cheek with your free fingers.

(3) It may be helpful to perform this procedure in front of a well lit bathroom mirror, cosmetic mirror or the FLOXITE. If the visual feedback is distracting, use tactile sensation only.

(4) Hold the VITAPICK applicator with one or two hands in a manner that is convenient. Do not rush.

  (a) **Touch the end of the tip to the tooth** right next to the gum line. See the following diagram.

  (b) Keep the tip perpendicular (parallel to the tooth axis or up and down) to the gum line. Slowly insert it into the gum crevice. This is generally painless. **Be careful not to pierce or penetrate the gum tissue with the end of the tip.** The greater pressure required to do this and pain will warn you to back off. Be gentle.

  (c) "Walk" or "hop" the end of the tip in the gum crevice. If there is a pocket the tip will "fall" in. Pockets can be wide or narrow. If you feel pain at any time withdraw the tip slightly or completely and try inserting again from a slightly different angle or location. For best results **keep the end of the tip in contact with the tooth.**

  (d) If at first you fail to enter a pocket, try again. Calculus, overhangs or ledges may hinder insertion. Gum inflammation may make insertion difficult and painful. An intrabony pocket as shown in the following diagram, is one which extends below the crest of the supporting bone (suprabony if it does not extend below). The surrounding bone may prevent the pocket from expanding which can make the insertion of the tip into the base of the pocket more difficult if not impossible.

  (e) Wiggle the tip gently while inserting it into the pocket. Do not apply too much pressure. Continue inserting the tip deeper. Wiggle and "explore" to find the base of the pocket. If the pocket has an irregular shape, is very narrow or the surrounding gum is inflamed, it can make reaching the base of the pocket difficult or painful.

  (f) Continue gently "wiggling" until you find resistance. This often indicates that you have found the base of the pocket. At this point

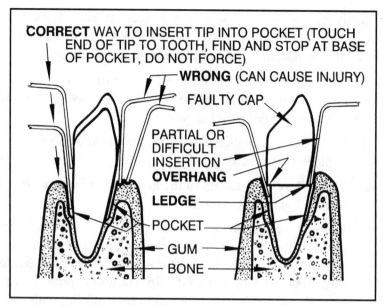

HOW TO INSERT THE TIP

do not exert any more pressure. It is important that you get close to the base, because the closer you deliver the solution to it the more likely it is that the deep bacteria is killed.

(g) The tip may be reshaped with your fingers to adjust the angle. Experiment! You may prefer to have two VITAPICKS, each with a tip that has a different angle.

(h) Push the plunger of the applicator to deliver the solution. If the end of the tip has reached the base of the pocket you may have to use additional pressure on the plunger to eject the solution. You may withdraw the tip slightly to allow the solution to flow easier. Experiment!

(5) Apply the equivalent of a drop or two of **antiseptic** or **antibiotic solution** at the base of the pocket.

(6) To be safe, at first work on only one pocket until you have mastered this procedure. Your inexperienced probing may irritate the gum and improper usage may cause infection. Follow the instructions step by step to avoid any problems.

(7) If the applicator was filled with antibiotics flush it out (fill and empty) once or twice with water.

PART X
ANTIBIOTICS

67. WHICH ANTIBIOTICS TO USE

Antibiotics are anti-infective agents of biologic origin. The primary antibiotic of dentistry is tetracycline. It is a broad spectrum antibiotic, effective against many bacteria but especially effective against anaerobic bacteria. Tetracycline and a few other antibiotics have consistently been shown to be very effective at eliminating gum infections.

1) **ACHROMYCIN** and **AUREOMYCIN** 3% tetracycline ointment are **nonprescription** antibiotics. Many drugstores stock it.

   (a) It is fairly viscous and may be applied with floss. See section 72(5).

   (b) When the means to safely liquefy it without greatly diluting it (so that it will flow through a thin gauge cannula) you may apply with the applicator.

   (c) If a nonprescription 2% to 4% tetracycline liquid becomes available then use it in the applicator.

(2) **Tetracycline** requires a **prescription** from a dentist or a physician. Ask for the 250 mg capsules, not tablets. Most drugstores stock it.

   (a) It can be mixed with water at 25 mg to 50 mg per milliliter of water which will yield a 2.5% to 5.0% tetracycline solution. You may dissolve the contents (250 mg) of the tetracycline capsule in 8 milliliters (a little less than two teaspoons) of water. The solution is delivered to the base of the pocket with an applicator. See section 74(4).

   (b) This yellow powder may be applied in tiny amounts to the gum crevice with floss or a toothpick. See section 72(6).

(3) If tetracycline is contraindicated for you, seek professional advice for alternatives. Other antibiotics (many in the tetracycline family) that have been used to treat periodontitis include: Achromycin 4% opthalmic tetracycline, amoxicillin, Augmentin, ciprofloxacin, clindamycin, doxy-

cycline, erythromycin, Keflex, metronidazole, minocycline, Myocin, penicillin, spiramycin, Terramycin.

68. LOCAL AND SYSTEMIC ANTIBIOTICS COMPARED

To treat gum infections antibiotics can either be applied locally (but not topically), taken orally or injected systemically. Below is a comparison on the local and systemic use antibiotics.

(1) In THE SMILE METHOD to treat infection, a tetracycline (or equivalent) solution is applied **locally**, in the gum crevice or pocket.

    (a) Applied this way, the concentration of tetracycline in the gum pocket is high enough to treat gum infection, yet this amounts to one thousandth of what one would consume systemically for the same effect.

    (b) Due to the tiny dosage used, the application of antibiotic in the pockets has fewer consequences than systemic dosing, Some improvement of a gum infection may be noticed as early as several hours after application.

    (c) It may take a few or several applications of tetracycline for severe or an abscess to subside. The initial application of antibiotics followed by periodic use of antiseptics combined with THE SMILE METHOD daily routine will considerably help to delay the recurrence of infection.

    (d) Annual or semi-annual preventive single or multiple dose application of an antibiotic solution to all pockets may be considered. More research is required to determine the safety of long term periodic use of locally applied antibiotics.

    (e) On my wish list is that someone develop and produce a low-priced, disposable, ready to use at home, pre-filled, antibiotic pocket applicator. It should be capable of dispensing the solution into the base of deep pockets the equivalent of one drop at a time.

(2) **Systemic** antibiotics are good for systemic infections or when localized application is not feasible. There are major objections to systemic use of all antibiotics. Some are listed below. Your dentist will asses the risk involved and the benefit that may be derived. The problems associated with systemic antibiotics cannot be completely ruled out for locally applied antibiotics in the case of (a) and (b).

(a) You may develop a sensitivity to a specific antibiotic. This sensitivity can cause you to have an allergic reaction next time it is used.

(b) Resistant strains of bacteria can develop rendering the antibiotic used ineffective. This may cause a superinfection, an infection by the resistant strains. Other antibiotics that are effective against the resistant strains will then have to be found.

(c) You may be overrun by non-susceptible organisms including fungi and bacteria, which may if pathogenic cause gum or other health problems.

(d) Taking tetracycline systemically takes one thousand times the amount to eliminate gum infection than does the application into the pocket as recommended by THE SMILE METHOD. Unfortunately the tetracycline reaches parts of the body that do not require it or may even be harmed by it.

(e) The systemic use of tetracycline and most of the other antibiotics may cause gastrointestinal problems including nausea, vomiting and diarrhea.

(f) Systemic antibiotics often upset the ecology of the normal flora necessary for health. To help rebuild the intestinal flora eat yogurt or take acidophilus supplements daily. Do this at least for a while after a course of systemic antibiotics.

(g) Dentists have prescribed tetracycline to be taken orally, 1 gm per day for up to fourteen days. Some tetracycline slowly ends up and accumulates around the pocket which usually eliminates the gum infection, at least temporarily.

69. VITAPICK AND ANTIBIOTIC FIBERS COMPARED

Time-release antibiotics, mostly tetracycline or metronidazole impregnated plastic fibers (bands, strips) are now approved for use in the USA by the FDA. Note the following:

(1) The fibers are periodically placed in deep pockets by your dentist to treat or prevent gum infections.

   (a) Long term frequent and periodic use of antibiotics is not generally recommended. Other anti-infective agents are being researched to replace the antibiotics.

      (b) You may experience some discomfort. The fibers are removed seven to ten days later. Experiments have been made using materials that slowly dissolve which may do away with the second visit.

      (c) Your dentist should inspect the site when he removes the fibers to ascertain that it is not infected. This is time consuming and expensive.

(2) It is uncertain how long the fibers or for that matter solutions will keep a pocket free from infection.

      (a) When treated with fibers, do you visit your dentist every time you suspect a site is infected?

      (b) The VITAPICK applicator may be used conveniently any time at home to deliver **antiseptics** periodically for prevention or upon the first sign of infection. You also have the added benefit of instant diagnosis with the absence or presence of stinging (when using salt and hydrogen peroxide). **Antibiotics** can be applied with the applicator if the antiseptic solution does not eliminate the infection. Using the applicator is thus safer to use and saves your time and money.

(3) Solutions and fibers have inherently different dispersion properties.

      (a) These fibers create "hot spots", within a pocket, where there is a high concentration of antibiotic and areas that may contain little if any. The "hot spot" is probably not dangerous though it may reduce effectiveness. This needs to be researched.

      (b) Antibiotic solutions when applied in the pocket are evenly diffused. It is the nature of all liquids to diffuse. The whole pocket is treated without creating a "hot spot".

(4) The fibers may not eliminate a periodontal abscess while proper use of the VITAPICK with antiseptic or antibiotic solutions can.

(5) If you lack manual dexterity and are unable to use the VITAPICK then ask your dentist to do so. Ask him to apply antibiotic solution in your pockets using these applicators or his subgingival irrigator/applicator. If he resists, then fibers may be your only non-systemic antibiotic alternative to treating deep pocket infections.

70. ANTIBIOTICS - SAFETY WARNING

Certain handling and usage precautions should be taken with antibiotics.

(1) **CAUTION:** Locally applied antibiotics should not be used as part of a long term daily, weekly or monthly routine preventive program. Use antibiotics only when other means have failed or are certain to fail to eliminate your gum infection. Ask your dentist to consider semi-annual or annual application. Systemic antibiotics should be taken **only** if they cannot be applied locally.

(2) It is very important that the balance of the oral bacteria most of which does not promote periodontitis and may actually promote oral health is not disturbed. To minimize this, perform the items listed below whether at home or at your dentist's office. During application of antibiotics into the pockets, using the VITAPICK or by other means, some solution will undoubtedly overflow into the oral cavity.

   (a) Blot the antibiotic solution that overflows with gauze, cotton ball or a facial tissue.

   (b) Some of the antibiotic which overflows may stick to the teeth. Look and remove excess by gently manual-brushing the effected teeth with water. Brush gums and tongue and rinse with warm water several times.

   (c) Visually check again to see if any tetracycline is still clinging to the teeth. Repeat blotting, brushing and rinsing if necessary.

   (d) Avoid swallowing the overflow that contains antibiotics.

(3) Once tetracycline is in solution, use it within twelve hours. If you are not sure how long an antibiotic is safe to keep in solution, dispose of it right after using it. Empty the unused portion in the drain. Never use antibiotics after the expiration date.

(4) Clean and remove the antibiotic residue from the measuring cup. To remove the antibiotic residue from the applicator, with tip in place fill and empty at least two times with water. Wash hands.

(5) **CAUTION:** Avoid contact with eyes.

(6) **CAUTION:** Pregnant women and those allergic to some antibiotics should use them only under a dentist's supervision.

(7) **CAUTION: KEEP ANTIBIOTICS, ALL DRUGS AND DANGER-OUS SUBSTANCES AWAY FROM THE REACH OF CHILDREN.**

(8) Read the leaflet accompanying the antibiotic (and all drugs) for contraindications, warnings, precautions and other details. If not enclosed in the box, ask your pharmacist for a copy or go to your local library and look it up in the PDR (Physician's Desk Reference) or other drug reference guide.

PART XI
TREATING GUM INFECTIONS

71. STATES OF GUM HEALTH & WHAT TO DO - OUTLINE

Gum infections will recur if you do not follow THE SMILE METHOD properly or slack off. Infection can recur because of bad health or for reasons that may not be obvious or understood. The various levels of gum health that you will encounter and what to do are listed below.

(1) There are no symptoms of infection. Your diagnosis has not found any sites to be infected. Some sites may be in remission. If you are fairly confident that **no pockets are infected** then continue following THE SMILE METHOD as you have been.

(2) **Asymptomatic** infections often go unnoticed. These usually low grade minor or chronic infections are difficult to detect. Some sites may be missed or misdiagnosed.

  (a) Since there are no symptoms to warn you, perform diagnostics periodically as a precaution. Check sites more often that experience tells you are more likely to be infected. See section 17.

  (b) Ask your dentist to see if he can locate any infected sites. See section 29.

  (c) **Shallow pocket** infections may be <u>prevented</u> by following THE SMILE METHOD daily routine. Often they can be <u>eliminated</u> by simply following the daily routine more attentively. See section 72(1) and (2).

  (d) To <u>prevent</u> reinfection, periodically (every three to fourteen days) use the VITAPICK applicator on all **deep pockets** or at minimum all troublesome sites. This will <u>diagnose</u> (see section 17(3) and (4)), <u>prevent</u>, <u>reduce</u> or <u>eliminate</u> these infections. See section 74(3).

(3) **Symptomatic,** suspect or sites diagnosed to be infected in **shallow pockets** (and gum crevice) can be effectively <u>treated by being more vigilant</u> with the tasks of THE SMILE METHOD daily routine and by various other means. See section 72.

(4) **Symptomatic**, suspect or sites diagnosed to be infected near or in **deep pockets** should be treated as follows:

    (a) Perform diagnostics on suspect and troublesome sites often and promptly when a site exhibits symptoms. See section 17.

    (b) THE SMILE METHOD daily routine can delay deep pocket infections from recurring but is not very good at eliminating them.

    (c) Treat suspect and diagnosed deep pocket infections accordingly. See section 74.

(5) A gum **abscess** and pockets that ooze out pus always indicates infection. It is likely that a deep pocket is near the symptom and should be treated promptly. See sections 74 and 75.

72. TREATING SHALLOW POCKET INFECTIONS

If when brushing or flossing, you see blood or notice other symptoms (e.g. bad odor, inflammation), probe to see if a deep pocket is located nearby. You may assume that this is as a shallow pocket infection if there are no deep pockets near the symptomatic site. First try (1) through (4) in any order, until the gum infection is eliminated. If that is not successful then try (5) or (6) and finally (7).

(1) **Floss** the infected site more <u>attentively</u> and more frequently, up to five times per day, but no more. If the site gets irritated or bleeding has not ceased in several days try (2), (3) or (4).

(2) **Irrigate or electric-brush** the infected site more <u>attentively</u> up to five times per day. Use a saturated salt and hydrogen peroxide solution, stronger than you usually use, up to 1.0%. Be gentle if the gum is inflamed, tender or sore. Be careful not to irritate it any more.

(3) **Tea Tree Oil** has penetrating and antiseptic qualities.

    (a) Use the lip and cheek retractor to aid in visibility and access.

    (b) With a clean towel or facial tissue, dry the gum around the infected site.

    (c) Dip a cotton swab in Tea Tree Oil or put a drop on fingertip and spread liberally on the gum near the problem site. Massage gum. Apply up to 5 times daily but stop if it is irritating. It has a sharp bitter flavor so it may take a while (if ever) to get used to it.

(d)　After the Tea Tree Oil is absorbed in two minutes or so, you may rinse mouth.

(e)　Tea Tree Oil may be found at many health food stores or purchased by mail-order.

(4)　Apply **baking soda** in the infected gum crevice:

(a)　To make this procedure easier, put on the lip and cheek retractor.

(b)　With your fingertip, rub and push soda into the space between the teeth from the tongue side and the outside of the infected site. Dry soda packs better than wet. Apply more soda. Press and squeeze as this may drive some soda into the crevice. This may be all that is necessary. If the infection is not eliminated by packing the soda try (c).

(c)　With your fingertip, rub a small amount of soda at the gum line near the infected site. Wet the soda with saliva to make slurry. Use floss to "sweep" the soda into the crevice. If the space between the teeth is narrow <u>insert the floss before applying soda</u>. "Sweep" several times. If floss breaks, and leaves a segment lodged in place, see section 62(11) and (12).

(d)　Avoid irritating the gum. Dry soda is abrasive, so be careful not to rub on gum as it may cause the gum to bleed. If stinging or inflammation worsens, stop. When finished you may rinse mouth thoroughly but very gently around the affected site to avoid removing the soda.

(5)　Apply **ACHROMYCIN** or **AUREOMYCIN** 3% tetracycline ointment in the gum crevice. This is a difficult procedure as the ointment is not easily controlled.

(a)　Review PART X - ANTIBIOTICS herein and read the leaflet enclosed in the package.

(b)　Apply a small dab of ointment on a clean surface or piece of paper.

(c)　Put on the lip and cheek retractor to increase visibility and accessibility.

(d)　With a clean towel or facial tissue, dry the gum and teeth around the infected site.

(e) Hold the floss (unwaxed) taut between two fingers and dip it into the ointment. Try to pick up approximately 1/2" (1.5 cm) of the ointment with the floss. You may also use the end of the tip from the VITAPICK or a toothpick to insert the ointment in the pocket.

(f) Insert the floss between your teeth with the adjacent "clean" portion. Move the floss covered with the ointment to the affected site. Using the floss try to pack or "sweep" the ointment into the gum crevice. Do this several times to make sure that some (only a tiny amount is required) ointment has been deposited in the crevice.

(g) Use facial tissue to remove any visible ointment. You may lightly brush teeth and tongue with warm water then gently rinse mouth to get rid of any residue. Do this several times and try not to remove the ointment from the crevice. Check to see if any excess ointment remains on teeth or gum. If so, repeat this sequence. See section 70(2).

(h) If infection has not cleared within three or four applications try (6) or (7) below.

(6) Apply **tetracycline** powder from capsules in the gum crevice.

(a) Review PART X-ANTIBIOTICS and the leaflet enclosed in the package.

(b) On a clean surface or a piece of paper, empty a little (approximately 50 mg) of the tetracycline powder.

(c) Put on the lip and cheek retractor to increase visibility and accessibility.

(d) With a clean towel or facial tissue, dry the gum area around the infected site.

(e) Hold the floss (unwaxed) taut between two fingers. Wet 1/2" of the floss with your tongue. Touch wet floss to the tetracycline, so that some adheres to it. Feed the adjacent "clean" floss between the "affected teeth". Move the floss with tetracycline attached over the affected site. Try to pack or "sweep" the tetracycline with the floss into the affected gum crevice. You may also try using a toothpick to maneuver the antibiotic powder into the crevice.

(f) It is difficult to know how much, if any, tetracycline was deposited in the gum crevice. Do not add any more as it is undiluted. Only a minute amount is required.

(g) Use gauze or facial tissue to remove any excess tetracycline. Lightly brush teeth and tongue with warm water then gently rinse mouth. Do this several times. Check to see if any excess tetracycline remains on teeth or gum. If so, repeat this sequence, but try not to remove any tetracycline from the crevice.

(h) If the infection has not been eliminated, it may mean that a pocket is located nearby. The base of a pocket cannot be reached by floss. Try (7) below.

(7) Apply an antiseptic or an antibiotic solution in the crevice or pocket with the VITAPICK in a similar manner as if treating a deep pocket infection. If treatment is not successful with the above methods, it may be that a deep pocket nearby is infected. Treat accordingly. See section 74.

(8) Massage gum especially around the infected site. Massage lightly at first. Use a finger or thumb. If it hurts you are being too aggressive. To save on time massage your gums while watching TV, walking or driving. See 74(2) and 17(8).

73. PERIODONTAL ABSCESS

A gum abscess (also known as a boiler or gum boil) is a sure sign of a severe infection. It may form as a result of a periodontal or a root canal infection (at the apex of the tooth) or combination of both. A root canal infection is caused by a dead or dying nerve and must be diagnosed and treated by a dentist. Only periodontal abscesses are discussed here. See section 96(2).

(1) A periodontal abscess is a localized inflammatory condition consisting of a cavity mostly filled with pus. It forms on the wall usually in deep pockets when the pus cannot adequately drain. This is a very critical time for the health of your gum and teeth. During this infection, pockets become deeper and additional supporting bone is lost in an accelerated manner.

(2) Bleeding or inflammation may precede the abscess, though often it forms without a warning.

(3) Dull throbbing, radiating pain usually is present during the acute stage

but mostly painless during the chronic stage. Sometimes it can be very painful.

(4) It feels like a spongy tender bump on your gums with a smooth and shiny surface. If the abscess is small or it is located between the teeth it may not be felt or seen.

(5) Pus may drain into your mouth giving you a foul breath and bad taste.

(6) It may be accompanied by malaise, fever and regional lymph node swelling.

(7) Not everyone with periodontitis gets it.

(8) Sometimes it goes in remission on its own.

(9) Periodontal abscess formation can be prevented and the duration shortened by following THE SMILE METHOD. See sections 74 and 75 that follow.

74. HOW TO PREVENT AND ELIMINATE DEEP POCKET INFECTIONS

Deep pocket infections range from low grade asymptomatic to severe with many symptoms. A severe infection may form an abscess. To minimize damage to gum and bone, always treat gum infections as early as they show symptoms or are diagnosed. Consider the following in the order listed:

(1) Take **vitamin C**.

    (a) At the very <u>first sign</u> of an infection especially if abscessed, take C-NBT dosage. See section 84.

    (b) If an abscess is especially pathogenic or the infection has spread systemically, your C-NBT level may increase abruptly, a little or by a considerable amount to over 50 grams per day. See section 85.

    (c) The dosage may seem excessive but if it helps the abscess from getting worse, then it beats visiting your dentist who may prescribe systemic antibiotics.

(2) **Massage** the gums.

    (a) By massaging your gums, you may detect anomalies that are the result of infection or an abscess. See section 17(8).

(b) If you locate an abscess, massage it <u>lightly</u> with a clean finger or thumb to increase circulation. This will permit the applied solution to diffuse, circulate and mix with the pus. Massage abscess before, during but not after using the VITAPICK.

(c) Massaging the gum may release pus and blood in the oral cavity. If so, rinse mouth.

(d) Start with a gentle massage and gradually increase the intensity in later applications.

(e) **CAUTION:** If you have any heart disorder, do not massage the abscess. There is the danger that some bacteria will be forced to circulate systemically.

(3) The **VITAPICK applicator with an antiseptic solution** is the <u>first method to use to eliminate deep pocket infections.</u> This is also the <u>best way to prevent deep pocket infections</u> from recurring, when used periodically.

(a) To make an antiseptic solution, fill the one ounce measuring cup with warm tap water and add approximately one teaspoon salt.

(b) Add 10 drops 35% hydrogen peroxide which will yield a 0.7% solution. Use 7 drops if irritating or 14 drops to increase effectiveness. Briefly stir to mix and to dissolve the salt. See section 107.

(c) Draw the equivalent of one or two drops of the solution into the VITAPICK. The drop technique allows you more control when using additional pressure to apply the solution at the base of deep pockets. You may find that fillilng the VITAPICK to capacity will save you time when applying the solution. See section 66(1).

(d) Locate the pocket and insert the tip. Eject the equivalent of a drop or two of antiseptic into the pocket. Applying too much solution, can sometimes cause pain, irritate and turn the gum temporarily white. See sections 65 and 66 and diagram near 66(5).

(e) If you notice any symptoms such as <u>bleeding or stinging</u> (see section 17(3) and (4)) gently repeat using the applicator up to five times daily until the bleeding stops and the stinging is hardly noticeable. To minimize stinging, at first use only a hydrogen peroxide solution diluted as low as 0.35%. Later you may increase the percentage and add salt. See 4(i) that follows.

(f) To **prevent** infections, at first perform this task every three days. Later to determine how often it should be performed, do it frequently enough so that no bleeding or little or no stinging occurs on subsequent tries. To be on the safe side do not exceed two weeks without repeating this task.

(g) You may use the VITAPICK with salt and/or hydrogen peroxide solution up to five times per day to help **eliminate** diagnosed (or suspect) gum infections or an abscess.

(h) Continue this task if you see improvement or until gum is healthy. If the infection worsens or does not diminish within five days, then try using colloidal silver in the VITAPICK. See section 37(4) and (4) which follows.

(4) If antiseptics did not previously, or you are sure that they will not eliminate the infection or abscess this time, then try the **VITAPICK with an antibiotic solution**.

(a) Flush out and clean the applicator before (and after) using it with an antibiotic solution. Pour 8 ml (a little less than two teaspoons) warm clean tap water in a clean one ounce measuring cup.

(b) Carefully twist open the 250 mg tetracycline capsule and pour contents into the water. The undissolved antibiotic will settle on the bottom. Stir to dissolve the antibiotic.

(c) Draw the equivalent of one or two drops of the solution into the VITAPICK. The drop technique allows you to use additional pressure to apply the solution at the base of deep pockets and minimizes the overflow. Draw in the solution from near the surface to avoid clogging the tip. See section 66.

(d) Massage abscess or affected site with fingers.

(e) Locate and insert the tip into the base of the pocket. Eject all of the solution into the pocket. Since you are filling the VITAPICK with only a drop or two of the antibiotic solution there will be a minimal overflow or spillage into the oral cavity.

(f) Use a facial tissue or gauze to absorb the excess.

(g) Rinse mouth often during application. Some antibiotic residue may remain on the tongue, cheeks or teeth giving a disagreeable taste. Brush teeth, gum and tongue with warm water to remove any antibiotic that may have stuck. Do this several times. See section 70(2).

(h) Locally applied it can overcome most gum infections with one, two or three applications. Apply it over one, two or three days.

(i) Antibiotics do not sting when applied in the pocket and thus do not alert you of an infection. However, if stinging is intense when using antiseptics you may at first use antibiotics.

(j) Make sure the infection has been completely eliminated. After the abscess has dissipated, apply up to six additional applications on alternate days. Apply four times on an infected pocket that did not have an abscess.

(k) Temporarily do not irrigate or floss the treated sites as this may dilute or remove some of the antibiotic from the gum crevice or pocket.

(l) Review section 70, ANTIBIOTICS - SAFETY WARNING.

(5) Sometimes, especially between widely spaced teeth, food may get wedged into the crevice or pocket. This may help promote an infection. To remove impacted food debris, try brushing, irrigating and flossing. If that does not work, use a metallic or plastic toothpick in combination with the VITAPICK (filled with antiseptic) to remove it.

75. TREATING AN ABSCESS

To eliminate the infection that forms an abscess, treat the pocket as previously suggested. Below is some additional advice on what to do if an abscess forms on your gums.

(1) You may use some of these methods to try to eliminate an abscess:

(a) Gently swish a very warm water salt solution (one tablespoon per cup) and direct it towards the abscess. Do this for one to two minutes every hour. This will help reduce inflammation.

(b) Some dentists suggest that you swish chamomile tea on the affected site. Chamomile tea has anti-inflammatory properties.

(c) My mother recommended that I include this prescription in this book. She used this method during the war years and claims it works. Well here it goes. Place some warm, moist and well boiled rice (medium grain, enriched?) of a thick consistency on the abscess and keep there for 15 to 20 minutes. Rinse mouth gently with warm water. Reheat rice and repeat three to four times daily. Start with a fresh batch of rice every day. Do this for several days until abscess shrinks or drains.

(d)   Brush gently and use a lower pressure setting when irrigating the abscess area, so not to further irritate and inflame the gum.

(e)   Do not repeat any of these methods if it irritates the affected site or your mouth.

(2)   Reduce your food consumption and keep your meals simpler by eating more fruits and vegetables in their fresh, whole and raw state. Avoid refined sugar!

(3)   During any type of health crisis the body is in need of extra restful living conditions. Rest more than usual. Decrease your work load and take a nap during the day. Go to bed earlier. Resting and sleeping is one way of conserving vital energy so that the body may better handle the present critical condition.

(4)   If this condition worsens, the infection may spread systemically. This may cause regional lymph node swelling, malaise and fever. People that have heart disorders such as carditis, rheumatic fever or rheumatic heart disease with heart valve damage, organic murmurs or a prosthetic heart valve are in additional danger during this crisis.

(a)   Your C-NBT level may rise a little or by a substantial amount, thus increase your C dosage to that level. See section 85.

(b)   See your dentist if you have a fever over 100°F (37.8°C) or have severe dental pain. He will more than likely prescribe a systemic antibiotic. Ask him to consider applying antibiotic solution in the infected pocket instead. If you were taking C-NBT, continue taking it as it will complement the antibiotic. C will help protect you against some of its harmful effects.

76. RELIEF OF PAIN DUE TO ABSCESS

A periodontal abscess can be very painful due to pressure it applies on the nerves. Inflammation whether caused by infection or trauma can also be painful. Pain will diminish as inflammation and infection are reduced. Try the following for relief:

(1)   Take C-NBT for its healing, anti-inflammatory and pain relief proper-
      ties. See section 84 and 85.

(2)   It is best to treat the cause of the pain rather than to try to cover it up
      with pain killers. For pain relief try:

      (a)   If you have a weak stomach try acetaminophen (TYLENOL or
            other brands). This is not anti-inflammatory, but will help reduce
            the pain.

      (b)   Try ibuprofen products (ADVIL or other brands) which are anti-
            inflammatory.

      (c)   Try buffered aspirin (BAYER or other brands) which is anti-in-
            flammatory. Do not follow the old practice of putting aspirin against
            the abscess as this does little if any good and can harm the gum
            tissue.

      (d)   Read attached label or leaflet enclosed in the package of pain re-
            lief products for warnings and cautions.

(3)   There are many over-the-counter topical pain killers available which
      contain benzocaine. Most of these are intended for temporary relief of
      dental pain. For more information read the label or ask your dentist or
      the pharmacist for advice.

(4)   Emergency pain relief consists of incision directly into the abscess and
      draining by your dentist. This quickly decreases pressure and relieves
      pain.

(5)   In an emergency when a dentist is unavailable and other means to re-
      lieve pain have failed try this:

      (a)   Sterilize a sewing needle preferably over the blue area of an open
            flame. Insulate the needle so not to burn your fingers.

      (b)   Let it cool.

      (c)   Prick the abscess (about 1/8" into it) to drain the pus. This in itself
            is not painful.

      (d)   The release of the pus will decrease the pressure will reduce the
            pain. Press abscess with finger or tongue to force out more pus.

      (e)   Rinse mouth with a warm salt water solution.

      (f)   Do not consume alcoholic beverages to block pain as it is often
            contraindicated by many pain relievers.

PART XII
SWASHING

77. WHY SWASH

You can use saliva to help keep your mouth clean, naturally. Swashing is derived from swish and wash. It is part of THE SMILE METHOD daily routine.

(1) Saliva has antiseptic properties that help sanitize your mouth.

(2) It will dislodge loose debris and plaque.

(3) It will improve breath odor and help moisten dry mouth if.

78. HOW TO SWASH

Swashing is an easy task to accomplish once you get the hang of it.

(1) Maneuver your tongue to the roof and bottom of your mouth. If you have not brushed, explore, locate and remove food particles with your tongue. All this will increase saliva flow. Experiment!

(2) Accumulate the saliva and swish it vigorously through your left teeth, then the teeth on the right side and then through the front teeth.

(3) Swallow your saliva (unless pus is present) as this is what you unconsciously do hundreds of times daily.

79. WHEN TO SWASH

Make a habit of swashing often. Swashing can be performed at any time.

(1) For sure swash if you forget to brush.

(2) Swash first thing in the morning for a fresher breath.

(3) Swash when driving, watching TV or walking.

(4) Swash even at night if you awaken with a dry mouth or throat.

(5) Good things can also be overdone so stop if it irritates your oral cavity.

(6) Though it may sound very loud to you, others will hardly notice.

PART XIII
SUPPLEMENTS

80. SUPPLEMENTS - OUTLINE

Vitamin and mineral deficiencies may develop for many reasons. Many of these deficiencies can produce symptoms of gum disease. Though deficiencies in some of these nutrients may cause gum problems it does not mean that supplementation will enhance the treatment of periodontitis. An improvement in your diet will usually eliminate the deficiency. If however the improved diet does not eliminate the deficiency, vitamin and mineral supplements may be tried. The following is the primary list of supplements that you may consider to help improve gum health.

(1) Vitamin C should be taken in conjunction with THE SMILE METHOD daily routine.

(2) Bioflavonoids may have a similar effect on gum health as vitamin C. There may exist some synergism between bioflavonoids and C. Vitamin C however does not require any additives.

(3) Vitamin B complex but especially folic acid may be helpful.

(4) Vitamin A as cod liver oil which includes vitamin D may be helpful.

(5) The essential minerals calcium and magnesium may help to stabilize bone loss.

(6) Coenzyme Q-10 may be helpful.

(7) Nutrition can be used to improve your health. There are many good books available on this subject.

81. VITAMIN C (ASCORBATE)

Much research into the health benefits of C supplementation has been performed. If you have any health problems I urge you to read the books written by Bland, Challem, Cheraskin, Newbold, Pauling, Sheffrey and Stone, which are listed in REFERENCES.

(1) At proper dosage, vitamin C is well known for its anti-cancer, anti-

glaucoma, anti-"colds", and pro immune system qualities. C also protects against arteriosclerosis and cardiovascular disease. This is the short list!

(2) Dr. Kalokerinos of Mosman, N.S.W., Australia is well known for his successful treatment of skin cancer using vitamin C ointment and for pain relief and life prolongation of other cancer patients with intravenous C. In a telephone conversation in early 1991 he stated that on average, adults should take 10 grams of C per day for health maintenance and prevention of cancer. The consumption of vitamin C supplements has spread globally and more physicians are now recommending it.

(3) Many studies have corroborated the benefits of vitamin C on periodontitis. Vitamin C supplementation has been shown to strengthen the periodontal membrane and connective tissue, reduce gum inflammation, inhibit bone resorption (shrinkage), aid in calcium absorption, diminish plaque formation, promote healing and helps stop gum bleeding.

(4) Vitamin C is essential for the formation of collagen, the protein matrix of bone (and teeth), the "glue" that holds the cells of your body together. Collagen fibers keep your gums attached to your teeth.

(5) By taking mega doses of vitamin C, using your tongue, you may be able to feel your gums tighten up around your teeth. The tightening of the gum around the pocket opening helps to keep out debris and bacteria. This also reduces tooth hypersensitivity.

(6) Scurvy is caused by a severe vitamin C deficiency. One prominent feature of this disease is that the gums bleed, teeth loosen and fall out. The same effects as periodontitis but at an accelerated rate.

82. VITAMIN C DOSAGE RANGE

The range of vitamin C dosing is listed below:

(1) You can not live without C.

(2) 10 mg (milligrams) of C cures most people of scurvy.

(3) 60 mg per day is the RDA (Recommended Daily Allowance for adults). This is easily obtained from fresh fruits and vegetables to maintain a good level of health.

(4) Mega dose 500 mg to 5 gm (grams) per day helps to prevent "colds" and to keep you healthy. Vitamin C dosage of over 1 gm can realistically only be obtained by taking supplements.

(5) If you have periodontitis, a daily C-NBT dosage can better help maintain you healthy and reduce gum infections. See section 84.

(6) The C-NBT level may rise with illness and gum abscess and so should the dosage. See section 85(1) and (2).

(7) The C-NBT level drops as health improves and so should the dosage. See section 85(3).

(8) During illness intravenous C may be prescribed at a higher dosage than the C-NBT level. See section 85(5).

83. VITAMIN C DOSING

Unlike most animals that produce their own vitamin C, and make a lot of it, the human body does not synthesize any. We need a lot more than our contemporary diet supplies. The amount of vitamin C you take daily determines its effectiveness. No two people are alike (different weight, health, genetics) in their vitamin C requirements.

(1) You should at minimum take a mega dose of C daily. Take 500 mg to approximately 50% of your average daily bowel tolerance level, which may be around 5 gm (5,000 mg).

(2) Daily dosage over 2 gm should be divided during the day. Do not take more than 5 gm at any one time. During illness you may dose many times during an hour but the total should not exceed 20 gm during this period.

(3) Vitamin C can be taken before, during or after meals, on an empty or full stomach. C capsules may be taken with any beverage.

(4) Dissolving the powder in water (or juice) is the preferred way to take vitamin C in doses over 5 gm per day. Capsules are a close second. I do not recommend that you take tablets because some may not dissolve properly and the binders used may spoil.

(5) Most people tolerate C less in the morning and the tolerance increases during the day and when asleep. If you encounter any problems experiment with timing.

(6) Make a note of every dose by simply writing a number to designate the grams. This will help determine your current daily dosage. When using powdered vitamin C (or for that matter all your supplements) write the date of first use on the bottle, so that when emptied, you may be able to calculate with accuracy your average daily consumption.

(7) For more consistent and accurate dosing of powdered C, use a measuring spoon. Check the label for weight equivalents. Depending on how fine the crystals are:

   (a) One level teaspoon of ascorbic acid is equal to 3.25 to 4.00 gm of vitamin C.

   (b) One level teaspoon of sodium ascorbate and the other ascorbates other than ascorbic acid is equal to 2.75 to 3.50 gm of vitamin C.

84. C-NBT DOSING

For many people, especially when ill, the C-NBT dosage is the ideal dosage. At these levels, vitamin C is virucidal and bactericidal.

(1) As a part of THE SMILE METHOD daily routine, I recommend that your dosage of vitamin C be approximately 90% of bowel tolerance, or an amount of C, Near Bowel Tolerance, from which I coin the acronym C-NBT. That is, if 10 gm give you diarrhea, then take about 9 gm.

   (a) Abdominal discomfort, abdominal growl, flatulence, gas, anal itch and/or soft stool often indicate that you are near bowel tolerance.

   (b) Diarrhea indicates that you have reached or passed the bowel tolerance level.

(2) Here are the steps to work out your daily C-NBT dosage. Only sodium ascorbate, calcium ascorbate and ascorbic acid are suitable for C-NBT dosing.

   (a) Start with 500 mg and gradually increase daily dosage. As your daily dosage increases to over 2 gm, divide the dosage during the day.

   (b) Trial and error is the only way to determine your C-NBT dosage. Time release C complicates C-NBT dosing by delaying feedback and should be avoided (it is OK to use for mega dosing). On my wish list is that someone come up with a practical fool proof method or a "litmus test" that will determine ones C requirement at any given time.

    (c)   If diarrhea does not pose any health risk to you, to gain experience, reach or slightly exceed your vitamin C bowel tolerance level.

(3)   Once you establish your C-NBT level, it stays fairly constant. A change in health may alter it. Over the years the level may very slowly rise as your system adjusts to your C dosage. Many adults can take 10 gm of C per day.

(4)   To test the effectiveness of C-NBT dosing on yourself try the following.

    (a)   As you increase the C dosage to C-NBT did your gums firm up and tighten up around the teeth? Did the amount of sites that bleed decrease? Was inflammation and other symptoms of disease reduced?

    (b)   Slowly decrease dosage until you stop completely. Do not change anything else in your routine. Give this test some time. If symptoms returned then you are fairly sure that vitamin C is effective.

    (c)   To double check the effectiveness of C, restart C-NBT dosing and see if your symptoms like bleeding and tenderness of gums are decreased or eliminated.

    (d)   The real test for C is how much it helps your periodontitis and overall health over the long term. Has your gum health improved? Are your days of illness fewer, shorter or less severe?

85. VITAMIN C DOSING DURING ILLNESS

Nutritionists and those practicing orthomolecular medicine often recommend vitamin (especially C) and mineral supplements above the RDA for therapeutic purposes. C-NBT is not the answer to all health problems, but as an aid in the prevention and elimination of gum infections it is very helpful.

(1)   Start C-NBT dosing on the first sign of worsening overall or gum health. Swollen or bleeding gums, bad breath, scratchy throat, coated tongue, swollen glands, runny nose, coughing, phlegm, body aches and low grade fever are some typical first signs of illness. What are your first signs?

    (a)   The C-NBT level may increase slowly or sharply as your overall health or gum health worsens. The C-NBT level may rise without any symptoms Though if your body cannot benefit from a higher

C dosage, you may get ill without the C-NBT level moving up.

(b) Increase intake (up to C-NBT level) regardless of how much C you normally take. In an effort to stay well or get well, you may have to take over 100 gm of C per day "chasing" your rising C-NBT level. Any dosage below your C-NBT level may be useless on acute illness.

(c) Due to a greater need, more of the vitamin C is absorbed. Less vitamin C then reaches the bowel, hence the greater tolerance for it. Titrate the vitamin C dosage between the amount which begins to make you feel better and the amount which almost but not quite gives you diarrhea. Not always easy to do!

(d) To avoid over shooting your bowel tolerance level (which may cause diarrhea), dose smaller quantities but more often. Dose even several times during an hour.

(2) Often, if vitamin C can be beneficial for an acute illness, the bowel tolerance for C will rise proportionally in relation to the severity of the illness. This will reflect the demand for C and thus what the dosage should be.

(3) As your health improves the C-NBT level will drop slowly or dramatically. Reduce C dosage proportionally.

(4) Your C-NBT level may be used as one barometer of overall health. For many people the color of their tongue reflects the state of their health. A coated white tongue may indicate illness. A really clean tongue reflects good health.

(5) Intravenous vitamin C has been used to treat various ailments and infections.

(a) It would be interesting to see how an intravenous C will deal with gum infections that may have spread systemically. If it turns out to be a successful treatment, it may be used as an alternative to systemic antibiotics which have risks and undesirable side effects.

(b) On my wish list is that someone develop and produce a safe, computer operated and monitored, portable intravenous C unit, which would free one from sitting at a clinic. Better yet, develop a form of vitamin C that when ingested can be tolerated by the bowel at higher levels.

(6) See a physician that is familiar with vitamin C therapy. Be aware though that most physicians and dentists are uninformed and more likely misinformed about C dosing.

86. VITAMIN C SIDE EFFECTS AND CAUTIONS

Vitamin C has some nuisance and minor side effects if you mega or C-NBT dose.

(1) Vitamin C dosage over what your body can use, reaches your bowel causing diarrhea. Prolonged or severe diarrhea is not good for health.

(2) Vitamin C in mega or C-NBT dosage, acts as a very mild diuretic (much milder than coffee). To combat this, drink more water (as thirst dictates).

(3) High dosage of vitamin C due partly to its diuretic quality may decrease blood pressure. Great if you have **high blood pressure** though you may want to avoid C as sodium ascorbate. If very **low blood pressure** causes you loss of energy or you are easily fatigued, add salt to your diet and/or consider taking C as sodium ascorbate.

(4) That prolonged high dosage of vitamin C may cause kidney stones is not well founded. In all my research I found no proof of this, so it either doesn't happen or it is a very rare occurrence. To be safe if you have a tendency to form urate stones see a physician that is familiar with vitamin C dosing. He can determine if the C should be acidic or alkaline to avoid this risk.

(5) If you consume high dosages of non-acidic vitamin C, it may be wise if you are prone to urinary tract infections to switch occasionally to ascorbic acid. The added acid will help prevent this infection.

(6) People who have a rare inherited ailment such as haemochromatosis, or sideroblastic anemia, both iron disorders, or thalassemia, should not take vitamin C supplements without a physician's supervision. The rationale is that C **increases iron absorption**, great for most of us but bad if this overloads your system with iron. There is however some evidence that C supplementation helps those with excess iron disorders in that C **normalizes iron absorption** thus helps to eliminate the excess iron.

(7) People that have kidney disease, sickle cell disease, or have a G-6PD

deficiency (up to 10% of black African-American males) and pregnant or lactating women should take C with caution. There exists some controversy in this area regarding how much if any C supplementation is safe and beneficial.

(8) Vitamin C, sometimes even at very low dosages (one orange) can cause false readings on a few clinical tests. For some tests, you may be required to refrain from taking vitamin C for up to seven days. Inform your doctor and lab technician of your C dosage. To get accurate results, alternate testing methods may be used.

(9) If you are taking a C-NBT dosage and are planning to stop or reduce it for any reason, do it gradually over two weeks. If you do not, the "rebound effect" may cause your body to react as if you have a C deficiency. This may lead to vitamin C deficiency symptoms. This has not been adequately demonstrated and may not always happen to everyone.

87. VITAMIN C - PURCHASING

Vitamin C which is also known as ascorbate comes in seven configurations: powder (or crystals), capsules, tablets, lozenges, chewable, syrup and liquid for injection or intravenous infusion. Vitamin C also is available in natural and synthetic, both being equally safe and effective.

(1) Ascorbic acid is the most common form of vitamin C. Ascorbic acid as the name implies, is an acid (pH 2.4), though a very mild acid and much milder than stomach digestive acids.

   (a) Avoid consuming ascorbic acid as a chewable (it often contains sugar), as a lozenge, in mouthwash, or dentifrices, because in these forms it can slowly etch the protective tooth enamel away.

   (b) If you ingest ascorbic acid in solution, rinse mouth afterwards to protect the tooth enamel.

   (c) If ascorbic acid gives you "heartburn", switch to non-acidic C.

(2) Sodium ascorbate because of its near neutral flavor and being non-acidic, has been my choice for some years now. Sodium may raise blood pressure and reduce tissue calcium in some people. This however needs to be better researched as the sodium in sodium ascorbate may differ in its effects. If you are on a salt-restricted diet, to be on the safe side, monitor your blood pressure to check if sodium ascorbate dosing raises it.

(3) Calcium ascorbate. The proponents of calcium ascorbate say that calcium in this form of C is well utilized.

(4) Magnesium ascorbate. Magnesium is essential for calcium utilization.

(5) Potassium ascorbate. The addition of potassium may lower blood pressure.

(6) Zinc ascorbate. The zinc may give an added boost to the immune system.

(7) Manganese ascorbate, Molybdenum ascorbate, Chromium ascorbate.

(8) Often Sodium ascorbate and calcium ascorbate are mixed in various ratios. You may also find all the buffered ascorbates (2) to (7) mixed together in various combinations. On my wish list is that someone market a blend of ascorbates that is palatable (if taken in solution), nutritious, economical, low or sodium free, that will not cause stomach distress.

(9) ESTER-C calcium ascorbate, is often sold with bioflavonoids in capsule form. The manufacturer claims that this patented form of vitamin C is more potent. It has a pH of 7.0. As a powder try ESTER-C sodium ascorbate which is very palatable and well tolerated when mixed in water. ESTER-C is more expensive than the regular C.

(10) Do not take the metal ascorbates in mega doses.

(11) There are some "hypo-allergenic" forms of C to try if you have allergy problems with it.

(12) Vitamin C is more economical if purchased in bulk, by the pound or kilogram. C has an excellent shelf life if kept dark and cool. Refrigeration is not required. Vitamin C loses its potency if stored moist or wet. To avoid adding moisture to the powder, dispense it with a dry spoon.

PART XIV
ADDITIONAL INFORMATION

88. THE SMILE METHOD COSMETIC BENEFITS

Below are some cosmetic advantages to THE SMILE METHOD:

(1) The primary cosmetic goal of THE SMILE METHOD is to prevent your gum line from receding further and thus maintain your great smile. Most people do not like to have long teeth as they feel it makes them look older or less attractive.

    (a) As more of the underlying bone that supports the teeth erodes, the gum recedes which exposes more and eventually all of the crown.

    (b) As the disease progresses it exposes the root.

    (c) Gum surgery which cuts back the gum, exposes even more of the root.

(2) Baking soda and hydrogen peroxide used in conjunction with the various tasks of THE SMILE METHOD daily routine will brighten and whiten dull stained teeth by removing stains if they are not too deep. Do not rush to have your teeth professionally whitened or bleached. Give THE SMILE METHOD from one month to six months to notice results.

(3) In THE SMILE METHOD ingredients that will stain the teeth such as chlorhexidine and rubber gum stimulators which may cause the gum to recede are not recommended.

89. HOW TO WHITEN YOUR TEETH

With all the money you save by using THE SMILE METHOD you may want to improve the appearance of your teeth. Below are several suggestions.

(1) The routine oral prophylaxis, (scaling and polishing) will help whiten your teeth. See section 27.

(2) If you still want brighter, whiter teeth, try brushing with PEELU tooth

powder. Just dip a moist toothbrush into the powder and brush. Rinse mouth with water after brushing. Avoid toothpastes that whiten teeth using strong abrasives. See section 37(1b).

(3) If you are not satisfied with the improvement you get from THE SMILE METHOD, then ask your dentist to whiten your teeth by chemically removing stains (with carbamide peroxide or hydrogen peroxide).

(4) Consider using over-the-counter whitening kits. Many kits are effective at whitening your teeth, though the safety issue needs to be better researched.

(5) If you are not satisfied with the results you get by following THE SMILE METHOD, or by professional whitening and you are unhappy with space between your teeth, there are several ways to correct this.

   (a) Your dentist can laminate veneers (fingernail or shell like) in the shade of white of your liking, to the front tooth surface which will cover these flaws. Ask your dentist if the veneers are made longer than the teeth they cover and if the added length will wear away the opposing teeth. If this is going to be a problem for you, ask your dentist to try to minimize it. Ask your dentist to be careful that the veneers do not restrict insertion of the VITAPICK tip.

   (b) A composite resin is brushed, shaped and polished directly to the tooth. It is less expensive and durable than veneers.

   (c) Materials and techniques are constantly being improved and prices are slowly dropping. Seek advice from your dentist regarding these techniques and alternatives.

90. CAPS AND BRIDGES

If you need a dental restoration such as a cap (crown, artificial crown) or a fixed bridge to replace a missing tooth, note the following items that have a direct bearing on periodontitis:

(1) Caps ideally should be indistinguishable in shape from the natural crown they replace.

   (a) Caps should not have overhangs or ledges. Faulty caps can irritate the gum and provide shelter for bacteria to multiply and accumulate. This can promote infection and make eliminating it more difficult. Overhangs and ledges can also make flossing or using the VITAPICK difficult or impossible. See diagram near section 66(5).

(b) Caps should not be bigger at the neck than the natural crown it will replace. Larger caps stretch the gum and make cleaning of the gum crevice difficult.

(c) Smaller caps allow debris to enter the crevice.

(2) Verify that flossing can be accomplished without any problem.

(a) Ask your dentist, to hold down the cap or fixed bridge with his fingers while you floss to check for overhangs or other problems, before permanent attachment. The floss should not snag or shred while inserting or removing from between your teeth.

(b) Check to see if you can easily feed the floss under the bridge using the floss threader.

(3) Some metal alloys used to make caps may irritate your gum. Ask your dentist for his advice.

91. HOW TO IMPROVE YOUR BREATH ODOR

Occasional bad breath due to the food consumed can be partially eliminated or covered up by various means. Bad odor may also originate in the gastrointestinal tract, lungs, throat or in the bacteria-trapping crypts of the nose. Some bad breath odor can be due to gum infection or an abscess. Some of the following suggestions may help eliminate this problem.

(1) By following THE SMILE METHOD you will in due time improve your breath odor automatically. You will find that a healthy mouth is odorless and does not require the use of flavored or scented mouthwashes. Morning breath can much be improved by the previous night performance of THE SMILE METHOD bedtime program.

(2) Brush, irrigate and floss. Rinse mouth thoroughly with water.

(3) Swash.

(4) Chew celery, carrots or sugarless gum.

(5) Try chlorophyll drops, aniseed and cardamon seeds.

(6) Try TIB, 100% pure essential flavor oils which come in many flavors (odors) in a tiny vial.

(7) MERFLUAN mouthwash concentrate which may also be used as a breath freshener. It contains no alcohol or fluoride.

(8) Try a low or non-alcoholic breath freshener or mouthwash. These may be found at your local health food store or drugstore.

(9) If bad breath persists then ask your dentist or physician for advice or see an ear, nose and throat specialist.

92. MOUTHWASH

Mouthwashes are used to improve bad breath (cosmetic) and/or fight gingivitis or periodontitis (therapeutic). Mouthwashes improve bad breath (halitosis) by the removal of food particles and loose plaque by the swishing action by chemically destroying some bacteria and by overpowering an offensive odor with a pleasant one. Try the following and see what works for you.

(1) The following formula for an odorless mouthwash will not mask any offensive mouth odor, but will safely help rid the mouth of some of the bacteria that causes it.

   (a) Add 7 to 14 drops of 35% food grade hydrogen peroxide to an ounce of warm water. You may rinse mouth then expectorate, but since you are using the food grade hydrogen peroxide, this is not necessary (unless you find it irritating). The hydrogen peroxide mouthwash effects will linger. Generally this formula should not be used on a daily basis for a long period or time.

   (b) A salt warm water solution also makes a good mouthwash. Add one or two tablespoons in a cup (8 ounce) of warm water. Swish in mouth or gargle with it. Expectorate and rinse mouth thoroughly with fresh water.

(2) You will find many non-alcoholic and fluoride-free mouthwashes at your local health food store.

(3) "I do not recommend commercial mouthwash to be used on a daily basis because many have a high alcohol content which has the potential to cause oral cancer," Dr. Wolner stated to me in a conversation we had in early 1989. Some mouthwashes contain as much as 28% alcohol.

   (a) Read label and select accordingly though the alcohol percentage is not always disclosed.

(b) Dilute high alcohol mouthwashes with water to decrease the risk factor.

(c) If you are using a high alcohol mouthwash to mask your breath odor, swish it around in your mouth only very briefly. Expectorate and rinse your mouth with water afterwards.

(d) **CAUTION:** Keep mouthwash out of reach of small children.

(4) Mouthwash does not penetrate into the gum crevice or pockets and thus is useless in treating infections there. Even when applied below the gum line with the VITAPICK most mouthwashes are still ineffective at eliminating gum infections. The following products have been advertised as being helpful in treating periodontitis.

(a) Chlorhexidine found in PERIDEX has been touted as being effective against periodontopathogens. PERIDEX contains 11.6% alcohol and the 0.12% Chlorhexidine is too low of a concentration to be effective. The other problem associated with this product is that it may stain your teeth.

(b) Sanguinaria found in mouthwashes (which may contain various amounts of alcohol) is not as effective as a saturated salt and hydrogen peroxide warm water solution.

(c) Avoid fluoride mouthwashes due to questions about their safety and effectiveness.

93. CHEWING GUM

Chewing gum helps moisturize the mouth, clean the teeth and exercise the facial and oral muscles. You may want to experiment to see which of the following brands best moisturizes your mouth and live up to the other claims made. The following products may be found at your local health food store or drugstore.

(1) BIOTENE dental chewing gum with enzymes and XYLITOL the natural sweetener that does not cause tooth decay and may stimulate saliva flow.

(2) KAL GUMGUM, it is sugarless and has all the vitamins and minerals that promote gum health.

(3) PEELU sugarless dental chewing gum.

(4) CHECK-UP plaque fighting gum.

(5)   XYLIFRESH sugar free gum with XYLITAL. It helps prevent plaque acids that can cause cavities.

(6)   TART-X chewing gum by FLOSS PRODUCTS Corp.

(7)   KAL-N-ZYME digestive enzyme chewing gum. Consider using this gum if you also have problems with digestion.

(8)   **CAUTION:** For those that have caps, inlays or fillings, chewing gum may dislodge them. See section 97(6).

94. LOZENGES

Zinc, folic acid and coenzyme Q-10 have been shown to be helpful in treating early periodontitis. These substances are used in lozenges. As they dissolve, some of these ingredients are absorbed by the gum.

(1)   Lozenges may be taken at the start of THE SMILE METHOD or when gum health deteriorates. Experience gained by trial and error will determine if lozenges are effective at preventing or decreasing the frequency of your gum infections. Try the following:

   (a)   SOLARAY makes a lozenge called DENTAL LIFE containing these ingredients with XYLITOL (a natural sweetener that does not promote plaque or tooth decay).

   (b)   LOZINCGES by KAL has zinc, vitamins A and C. Rinse mouth soon afterwards as it contains fructose.

(2)   People who have a peptic ulcer or who get a stomach ache when consuming zinc may slowly dissolve one zinc lozenge in the mouth approximately a half hour before a meal.

(3)   Under no circumstance should you sleep with lozenges in mouth.

95. TOOTHPICKS

Receding gums and widening space between teeth due to periodontitis, make it easier for food particles to accumulate between teeth. Do not substitute toothpicks (interdental cleaners) for floss. When floss is unavailable and a toothbrush will not do, use a toothpick.

(1)   Plastic toothpicks are best. They are quite pliable, will not crack or splinter. Plastic toothpicks are economical and generally reusable and are easily carried in a pocket or purse. I recommend that you try the following products.

(a) The PROPICK dental cleaners by ARMOND is a well designed plastic toothpick that can reach and remove food particles from the tightest space.

(b) The ROTA-POINT interdental cleaners by PRO-DENTEC have a well designed long narrow point that can be used to remove food particles from the tightest space.

(c) The PRO APPROVED has a well designed base with a straight and angled pick for really hard to reach spaces.

(d) The PLAC-PIK by PREVENTIVE DENTISTRY PRODUCTS, INC., is a green toothpick with the longest point which is textured to remove food particles.

(2) Try the T-PIK (keychain size) or ORAPIK (pen size), which are reusable metal toothpicks with protective covers. They are great at getting into tight spaces. The metal is not very flexible so use with caution. Avoid scratching the teeth.

(3) As a standby there are the round and flat wooden toothpicks, finger nails, twig, match book cover and business card to use. Use them but do not make a habit of it.

(4) There are several products that look like picks and are made of wood, rubber or plastic but are designed primarily to stimulate and firm up the gum. They are time consuming to use and may not be effective at treating periodontitis. Their daily use may cause the gum to recede.

96. WHAT TO DO ABOUT HYPERSENSITIVITY

A receding gum line and gum surgery expose all the crown and more of the root. The root of the tooth does not have the enamel insulation which covers and protects the crown. This may lead to hypersensitivity or tooth pain or discomfort due to the exposure to hot, cold, sweet, sour or salty foods and drinks, hydrogen peroxide or contact with toothbrush, floss, toothpick, or metallic probe. This can be temporary or last for many years. Swish cold or warm water in mouth to pinpoint sensitive spots and mark them on your tooth chart which you may show your dentist. If the pain becomes distracting or debilitating you may want to try the following home-care ((1) to (3)) or professional remedies:

(1) Avoid the items that cause discomfort or pain.

(2) Tooth sensitivity can increases for various reasons.

(a) A tooth can become more sensitive near an infected pocket. Follow THE SMILE METHOD to eliminate the infection. Note that cold water is colder in winter which makes hypersensitivity more noticeable. This may falsely lead you to believe that your gum health worsens then.

(b) A tooth may hurt when you drink warm beverages while cold ones bring relief. The tooth may also darken. This may be due to the decay of the tooth nerve (root canal). Call your dentist for advice.

(3) Brushing with DENQUEL, Original SENSODYNE, Mint SENSODYNE, BUTLER PROTECT, THERMODENT or PROMISE toothpastes may take two weeks to desensitize the hypersensitive teeth. Discontinue if you notice any side-effects.

(4) A thorough scaling by your dentist removes the calculus around the gum-line. This may reduce or eliminate tooth hypersensitivity.

(5) Daily rinsing on a temporary basis with a 0.5% stannous fluoride mouthwash may help.

(6) Application of sodium fluoride gel or calcium hydroxide derivatives on the sensitive tooth may help.

(7) BUTLER PROTECT or SENSODYNE Sealant Dentin Desensitizer (liquid) may be brushed on painlessly by your dentist. Partial or total relief is immediate in most cases and may last for up to six months.

(8) The DESENSITRON II or LIFE-TECK may be used by your dentist to apply 2% sodium fluoride solution using iontophoresis. This is painless and is partially or totally effective instantly in most cases.

(9) A bonding agent to the offending area may be applied by your dentist. This is painless and is partially or totally effective immediately in most cases.

(10) As the very last resort if the pain is persistent and disabling, your dentist may recommend removal of the tooth nerve (root canal).

97. HOW TO IMPROVE YOUR DRY MOUTH

There are several ways to increase saliva flow or to add moisture artificially.

(1) Keep a glass of water nearby (even at bedside) and sip often. Keep a little water in your mouth for as long as you can. If dehydration is a

problem, drink more water (six to eight glasses) during the day.

(2) Swash often but gently.

(3) Breathe in and exhale from nose or try inhaling through nose and exhaling through mouth to conserve moisture in the mouth. If you are having trouble breathing in through the nose due to congestion, then try taking C-NBT. Vitamin C at high dosages acts as an antihistamine and may help reduce or clear up your nasal congestion.

(4) Eat raw vegetables especially carrots and celery. Their high fibre content requires more chewing which stimulates saliva flow. Chewing also strengthens the teeth, gum and the jawbone. Their high water and nutrient content are also very beneficial.

(5) In low humidity areas or on low humidity days, use a humidifier. You may want to humidify only your bedroom when asleep, since that is when most mouth breathing is done. I recommend a hot steam humidifier, as they are inexpensive to buy. Steam is created by boiling the water. This is purified water and perfectly safe to inhale. It will not dust up your house and lungs like some other types of humidifiers. I do not have any brand name recommendations. Find one that is easy to maintain.

(6) The XENEX is a flexible plastic ball with a recessed track that you can chew for a long time to help saliva flow. It will not dislodge amalgams. It also cleans teeth and massages the gums.

(7) Chew sugarless gum when your mouth is dry.

(8) Suck on sugarless lozenge or candy. The sucking will increase saliva flow.

(9) Try CAMOCARE Throat Spray (sold at health food stores). It freshens and lubricates mouth, soothes throat and gums.

(10) Try ORALBALANCE Long Lasting Moisturizing Gel, made by the same people that make the BIOTENE toothbrushes. Also consider trying OREX, XEROLUBE, SALIVART and MOI-STIR which are sold over-the-counter.

(11) Brush with BIOTENE Dry Mouth Toothpaste especially before retiring for the night.

(12) Avoid alcoholic and sugared beverages, caffeine, smoking, salty, spicy and acidic foods.

(13) Ask your dentist for advice or see an ear, nose and throat specialist.

98. HOW TO IMPROVE YOUR HEALTH

There are many health philosophies and disciplines. It is beyond the scope of this book to discuss all of them. For details, I urge you to read some of the many good books on health that are available. I believe in the holistic approach, which treats all of the body and the mind (psyche, spirit or soul), not just the parts. The second meaning of holistic which I also subscribe to is the use of the safest and most effective concepts of the many health disciplines and philosophies. This is a summary of what I found noteworthy in my research.

(1) If you have all your teeth, you have 32 permanent teeth. They should last you a lifetime.

   (a) The loss of a tooth, due to periodontitis or other causes is very injurious to health.

   (b) The domino effect applies here. Do everything to avoid tooth loss. A missing tooth weakens neighboring teeth and so on down the line. As teeth are lost the stomach suffers, then the intestines, then nutrition and so on, until you slowly feel more sluggish and health problems appear.

   (c) The "everything" that you do to improve gum health to save your one, two or more teeth may not only prevent the domino effect but also improve your overall health.

(2) Taking vitamin C especially at a higher dosage, is the simplest way to help improve or maintain health.

(3) The ideal diet for the adult human organism can be expressed very simply in a three word summary. Remember these three words at every meal, better yet, before every meal, and check to see if the food you are eating falls under the category of all three words or at least two. The three words are:

   (a) **Whole** (unaltered). Whole as applied to the ideal diet means the food is in its natural, unprocessed state. Good examples are fruits, vegetables and nuts. Bad examples are white flour and all white flour products.

(b) **Raw** (fresh and ripe). Raw means that the food has not been altered by heat, the process of cooking. Good examples are raw vegetable salads and fresh fruit salads. Bad examples are cooked vegetables especially overcooked vegetable soups.

(c) **Plant** (fruits, vegetables, nuts and seeds). Plant food means that the original source of the food is from the plant kingdom.

(d) SUMMARY: Increase the consumption of fresh, ripe fruits; in fact, make a meal out of them. Eat fresh vegetables, salads (with little or no dressing). Eat an apple or carrot before or after lunch or supper. The more you improve your eating habits, and try to attain the "ideal diet" the better off you will be. The improvement of your health may be felt immediately but more likely you will notice the change and appreciate it in the years to come.

(4) Pick your proteins wisely.

(a) The best sources for protein are raw nuts, seeds, seed sprouts, avocados and ripe olives because they are loaded with nutrient and do not have the problems associated with animal products. None of the nutrients are lost to processing.

(b) Try legumes, brown rice and whole grain products.

(c) Though plant proteins are incomplete, by eating a variety of protein foods you can accumulate and use them as if they were complete.

(d) Strict vegetarians may develop a B-12 deficiency. This may take years to become evident, so as a safety precaution, supplement a diet that lacks animal products with vitamin B-12.

(e) If you can, eliminate red meats or at least try to consume smaller portions. Switch to chicken and especially seafood (steamed best, fried worst), yogurt or cheese (especially cottage cheese) for protein.

(5) Avoid sugar like the plague it is and foods that list sugar (or sucrose) as an ingredient. Besides encouraging plaque growth it is bad for mental and physical health.

(6)   Avoid consuming additional salt especially if you have high blood pressure. Consider adding salt to your diet if your blood pressure is very low and you are feeling run down. Before buying packaged food read the nutrition and ingredient labels. Salt may be listed as sodium chloride.

(7)   A good juicer can extract much of the juice from raw vegetables or raw fruit. A juicer can be rather expensive initially, but when you amortize it over the many years of use, it comes out to a few nickels per day. Factor in the money you will save through lower medical costs and thus it becomes profitable to own.

    (a)   Though this food is altered, it is altered without heat. Carrot and celery and other vegetable juices are loaded with nutrients. Try diluting the juice with water.

    (b)   Drink slowly and mix with your saliva before swallowing.

    (c)   Drink juices in moderation, as chewing raw vegetables and fruits is better for dental health than juicing them. Substitute juices for soda pop, coffee and junk food.

    (d)   Read some of the many good books available on the health benefits of fresh juices.

(8)   If you are over 35 years of age, consider eating higher fiber foods or taking fiber supplements.

    (a)   If one recalls from Greek Mythology: The moon Goddess Hecate fed dandelions to the hero Theseus, giving him power to kill the notorious Minotaur, a half-man, half-bull monster, who devoured young men and maidens. Theseus probably got his strength from the dandelion's iron content (or was it the fiber?) which has a little more than spinach; and everybody knows what eating spinach did for Popeye. Modern day Greeks prepare dandelions (endives or spinach) by boiling them and adding some olive oil (isn't Popeye's girlfriend named Olive Oyl?) and lemon over it. They eat this along with whole wheat bread, feta cheese and olives. As a side dish, or as a main dish twice a week, it will provide the best fiber and roughage that nature can offer.

(b) If on the other hand you decide to take fiber supplements you will have a big variety to choose from. They are all good, but some are better formulated. Some have added lactobacillus acidophilus to help improve colon health. Experiment to see which one and what dosage works best for you.

(9) Exercise five times per week, at least half an hour per day. Get your muscular and cardio-vascular system in shape. Modern health specialists say exercise may be even more important than diet to maintain health. There are so many good books on this subject that I am not going to mention details.

(10) For good health you should also have a positive attitude toward yourself, people and life in general. Think positive thoughts about yourself and environment. Plan your days, weeks, your life in a positive and creative way.

(11) This may sound silly, but nevertheless it works. LAUGH! Laughing is aerobic. Laugh as many times as you can even if you have to force yourself. Children laugh 400 times a day. Laugh out loud (in private) in your auto, washroom or wherever you feel comfortable. Laugh the gloomy feelings completely out of you.

(12) When reading the book every time you see "SMILE" I want you to smile. Every time you see someone smiling, smile back. It is contagious, so spread it around. If they are not smiling, smile at them anyway. It does not cost anything. SMILE, SMILE, SMILE! Be happy! Let the life-force energize your total being. Hopefully the results attained by following THE SMILE METHOD will put a SMILE on your face.

PART XV
GAUGING PROGRESS

99. GAUGING SHORT TERM PROGRESS

It is important for you to know what progress you are making in controlling your periodontitis. Monitor your dental health regularly. Knowing what works and what doesn't will help you modulate your routine. To determine your progress, review your records and notes you have taken. Go through the list below to see if you have made these improvements.

(1) Bleeding when brushing, flossing or irrigating has stopped. It may take ten to thirty days from the day you start THE SMILE METHOD.

(2) Tooth mobility will be slightly less, or in some instances considerably less. Mobility may be reduced even on teeth that were considered "hopeless" or were ready for extraction.

(3) There will be no sign of pus and periodontal abscesses will not form. If it occurs, abscess formation will not last long, due to your improved health and the "know how" to eliminate them.

(4) If there is pain, depending on the cause, will be diminished or eliminated.

(5) Gums will feel tighter and firmer.

(6) Mouth odor will be normal unless you have other health problems.

(7) The color and texture of the gum will improve.

(8) The most sensitive indicator of infection is stinging.

   (a) If you do not have any obvious symptoms, stinging when applying salt or hydrogen peroxide solution to the base of the pocket very likely indicates infection.

   (b) The absence of stinging may indicate no infection is present or that the salt solution has not reached the base of the pocket.

(9) SUMMARY: The damage caused by periodontitis cannot be reversed. Most of the time you will be without symptoms. Your self-diagnosis

and your dentist's diagnosis of questionable sites will more often be negative.

100. GAUGING LONG TERM PROGRESS

Some parts of the dentition deteriorate very slowly and thus detection and recognition of any problems takes longer. Periodic monitoring and good record keeping are essential for gauging long term progress. Take notes frequently of setbacks and progress. Notes need not be long to be useful. Do not rely on memory. Fill out the READER'S HEALTH SURVEY before starting treatment. Use this and your dentist's records as of the latest visit as the base for future comparisons.

(1) If THE SMILE METHOD is helping you, shallow and deep pockets will stop getting deeper. Pocket depth may be reduced slightly. Annually or at maximum biannually ask your dentist to measure all your pockets. Troublesome and deep pockets should be probed more often. He should record the depths for comparative purposes. Keep in mind that pocket depth measurements are not consistent and will fluctuate, so use them only as a rough guide. See sections 25(1), 25(3) and 28(2).

(2) The deterioration of the supporting bone will be stopped or substantially slowed down. This is hard to quantify though the new digital imaging technology can help in this respect. See section 28(4).

(3) Tooth exposure due to gum recession will stop increasing. Dentists do not do this but you should measure tooth exposure of front teeth. See diagram near section 20(4).

(a) Stand in front of a well lit magnifying mirror with the lip and cheek retractor in place and a periodontal probe in hand. You may recruit a family member or friend to help.

(b) Place the calibrated tip at the center line of one tooth. Measure the distance from the chewing surface to the gum line. Record the measurement. Continue measuring the other top seven teeth and the bottom eight.

(c) This will establish the baseline measurement of your gum line. All future measurements will be compared to this. The more accurate your measurement is the more reliable your analysis will be.

101. IF THE SMILE METHOD HAS NOT HELPED YOU

After gauging your short term and long term progress, and the results were unsatisfactory read below.

(1) If you do not have adult periodontitis or it is atypical, there are complications, or your case is refractory (about one out of twenty of all cases) THE SMILE METHOD may not benefit you. These cases are outside the scope of this book. It may be a good idea to review your diagnosis with your dentist though any atypical aspect of your periodontitis may not be easily revealed.

(2) If your overall health is extremely poor, you must deal with your whole organism to recover health at all levels. Following THE SMILE METHOD will only give you partial success until you regain your health.

(3) If you do not visit a dentist THE SMILE METHOD cannot be fully implemented and thus will not be fully effective. If your dentist does not cooperate and does not assist you to implement THE SMILE METHOD, do not expect total success. Without his assistance you will not be able to properly implement it.

(4) After gauging your progress, and you find that your gum health is not noticeably better within two months, consider that you may not be following the routine properly. Review book, and especially parts that may be relevant to you. Modulate your routine and monitor gum health frequently. Experience will help your fine tune and tailor THE SMILE METHOD to your needs.

(5) If at the end of three months you see no improvement in your gum health, stop THE SMILE METHOD. If whatever you are doing is not making you better, it may be hurting you, because maybe you should be doing something else. All that you have done has not helped so try something different. I urge you to contact various health organizations. Call or see your dentist, physician or health practitioners of the various disciplines and philosophies. See section 23, FINDING A DENTIST.

PART XVI
MOTIVATE - INFO - SURVEY

102. STAY MOTIVATED

THE SMILE METHOD is only as good as you are good at following it. Follow it everyday and you will be rewarded.

(1) This is how I motivate myself.

    (a) On the positive side I remind myself of the smile I will maintain and the teeth that I will save if I continue following THE SMILE METHOD.

    (b) On the negative side I motivate myself by reminding myself of the dire financial, painful and cosmetic consequences of slacking off.

(2) The only time you fail is when you stop trying.

    (a) If you give up and elect to have surgery you may end up with a more demanding and time consuming maintenance program.

    (b) If you give up and do nothing to improve your gum health, then you will lose your teeth one at a time.

(3) Since you have read this far, then you must have enough motivation to get started! When you see improvement in your gum health it will encourage you to continue!

(4) The final wish on my wish list is that your desire to improve your gum health will motivate you to follow THE SMILE METHOD daily and that you are as successful with it as I am.

103. STAY INFORMED

As all branches of science, technology and medicine advance, it is advisable that you keep yourself informed of such developments.

(1) I recommend that you fill out the READER'S HEALTH SURVEY and file along with your dental records and notes. This is important so that

in the future when the need arises you will have this valuable information available to refer to.

(2) You may want to send me a filled out copy of your READER'S HEALTH SURVEY. All medical information will remain confidential.

(3) I will try to keep you informed of any advancements in the nonsurgical treatment of periodontitis. I can be reached through Albrite Inc. For address see section 19(1).

104. READER'S HEALTH SURVEY

(1) Date: _____ - _____ - _____

(2) Name (Last, First): _____

(3) Address : _____

(4) City, State and Zip (Country): _____

(5) Phone No.: (_____) _____ - _____

(6) Age: _____ Birthdate: _____ - _____ - _____

(7) Sex: M -- F

(8) How would you rate your health? EXCELLENT--GOOD--FAIR--POOR

(9) What are your major health problems?_____

_____

(10) Are you taking any medication? YES--NO--WHICH: _____

(11) Do you have any allergies? YES--NO--TYPE: _____

(12) How many "colds" per year do you get? NONE, 1, 2, 3, 4, ____

(13) How many days do they last? 1, 2, 3, 5, 7, 10, 15, 20, ____

(14) Do you have bad breath? (check!)
     NEVER--RARELY--OFTEN--ALWAYS

(15) Do your gums bleed spontaneously?
     NEVER--RARELY--OFTEN--DAILY

(16) Do your gums bleed when brushing?
     NEVER--RARELY--OFTEN--ALWAYS

(17) Do your gums bleed when flossing?
     NEVER--RARELY--OFTEN--ALWAYS

(18) Have you noticed any pus around some teeth?
     NEVER--RARELY--OFTEN--ALWAYS

(19) Does your floss occasionally get snagged or shred at some sites? Y--N

(20) Are your gums spongy to the touch?

     NEVER--RARELY--OFTEN--ALWAYS

(21) Do you get a gum abscess? NEVER--RARELY--OFTEN

(22) Do you feel pain when chewing?
     NEVER--RARELY--OFTEN--ALWAYS

(23) How many of your teeth are loose? (check!)
     NONE--ONE--SOME--MANY--ALL

(24) Have spaces between teeth widened? YES--NO

(25) Has your gum line receded? NO--A LITTLE--A LOT--CANNOT TELL

(26) What color are your teeth?
WHITE--LIGHTLY STAINED--HEAVILY STAINED

(27) Are some of your teeth sensitive to: HOT DRINKS--COLD DRINKS-
-SWEETS--SALT--HYDROGEN PEROXIDE--CHEWING PRESSURE-
-FLOSSING--TOOTHPICK--METALLIC PROBE

(28) How many teeth do you have now? (Count them!) 32, 30, 28, _____

(29) How many teeth have you lost? 1, 2, 3, 4, _____

(30) How many teeth have been extracted? 1, 2, 3, 4, _____

(31) How many due to: CAVITIES _____ PERIODONTITIS (loose) _____
CROWDED ARCH _____ OTHER:_____

(32) How many teeth have you replaced? FIXED BRIDGES _____ PAR-
TIAL UPPER DENTURES _____ PARTIAL LOWER DENTURES ___
FULL UPPER DENTURES _____ FULL LOWER DENTURES _____

(33) Every how many months do you visit your dentist? 1, 2,3, 4, 6, 12, _____

(34) When did you last visit your dentist? _____ - _____ - _____

(35) What transpired? _____

(36) Has your dentist diagnosed adult periodontitis? Y--N What year? _____ .

(37) What stage is it in? EARLY--MODERATE--ADVANCED

(38) How many mm (millimeters) deep is your deepest pocket? _____ .

(39) Did your dentist recommend gum surgery? YES--NO

(40) Did you have gum surgery? YES--NO

(41) Are you satisfied with the results? YES--NO

(42) If not, why not? COST--PAIN--APPEARANCE--HYPERSENSITIVITY-
- LONG MAINTENANCE ROUTINE--HEALTH--OTHER_____

(43) Do you plan to follow THE SMILE METHOD? YES--NO

(44) If you are already following THE SMILE METHOD, has your
periodontitis improved? MUCH--LITTLE--NONE--WORSENED

(45) How long have you been following the SMILE METHOD?_____ .

(46) On a separate sheet make brief remarks about your present and past health,
gum health, problems, progress and setbacks, gum surgery, your dentist,
comments and criticism about THE SMILE METHOD and this book.

PART XVII
TABLES

105. DILUTING 35% FOOD GRADE HYDROGEN PEROXIDE (BY PARTS)

The solutions that may be used as part of THE SMILE METHOD are in bold. If you add one part 35% food grade hydrogen peroxide (H_2O_2) to:

100 parts water you will end up with a 0.35% H_2O_2 solution.

87 parts water you will end up with a 0.4% H_2O_2 solution.

70 parts water you will end up with a 0.5% H_2O_2 solution.

58 parts water you will end up with a 0.6% H_2O_2 solution.

50 parts water you will end up with a 0.7% H_2O_2 solution.

44 parts water you will end up with a 0.8% H_2O_2 solution.

39 parts water you will end up with a 0.9% H_2O_2 solution.

35 parts water you will end up with a 1.0% H_2O_2 solution.

29 parts water you will end up with a 1.2% H_2O_2 solution.

23 parts water you will end up with a 1.5% H_2O_2 solution.

106. DILUTING 3% HYDROGEN PEROXIDE (BY PARTS)

The solutions that may be used as part of THE SMILE METHOD are in bold. If you add one part 3% U.S.P. hydrogen peroxide (H_2O_2) to:

8 parts water you will end up with a 0.35% H_2O_2 solution.

5 parts water you will end up with a 0.5% H_2O_2 solution.

3 parts water you will end up with a 0.75% H_2O_2 solution.

2 parts water you will end up with a 1.0% H_2O_2 solution.

1 part water you will end up with a 1.5% H_2O_2 solution.

107. DILUTING 35% FOOD GRADE HYDROGEN PEROXIDE (BY DROPS)

The solutions that may be used as part of THE SMILE METHOD are in bold.

If you add 1 drop of 35% H_2O_2 to 1 oz. of water you will end up with a 0.07% H_2O_2 solution.

If you add 5 drops of 35% H_2O_2 to 1 oz. of water you will end up with a 0.35% H_2O_2 solution.

If you add 7 drops of 35% H_2O_2 to 1 oz. of water you will end up with a 0.5% H_2O_2 solution.

If you add 10 drops of 35% H_2O_2 to 1 oz. of water you will end up with a 0.7% H_2O_2 solution.

If you add 14 drops of 35% H_2O_2 to 1 oz. of water you will end up with a 1.0% H_2O_2 solution.

If you add 21 drops of 35% H_2O_2 to 1 oz. of water you will end up with a 1.5% H_2O_2 solution.

108. WEIGHT AND VOLUME EQUIVALENTS OF FLUIDS

ml (milliliter) = cc (cubic centimeter) = gm (gram) = 1000 mg (milligrams)

1 drop = 60 mg

1t (teaspoon) = 80 drops = 5 gm = 5 ml = 1/3T = 1/6 oz.

1T (tablespoon) = 240 drops = 14 gm = 14 ml = 3t = 1/2 oz.

1 oz. (ounce) = 480 drops = 28 gm = 28 ml = 6t = 2T

8 ounces = 1 cup = 1/2 pint

16 ounces = 2 cups = 1 pint = 1/2 quart = 1/8 gallon

32 ounces = 4 cups = 2 pints = 1 quart = 1/4 gallon

128 ounces = 4 quarts = 1 gallon

REFERENCES

Adams R, Murray F. *Improving Your Health with Zinc.* Larchmont Books, New York, 1978.

Allen DL, McFall WT Jr, Jenzano JW. *Periodontics for the Dental Hygienist.* Lea and Febiger, Philadelphia, 1987.

Amigoni NA, Johnson GK, Kalkwarf KL. The use of sodium bicarbonate And hydrogen peroxide in periodontal therapy: a review. *JADA* 114:217-221, Feb. 1987.

Anderson GB, Smith BA. Periodontal probing and its relation to degree of inflammation and bleeding tendency. *J Western Soc Periodont/Periodont Abs* 36(3):97-241, 1988.

Annotations. The International Dental Health Foundation, 1982 to 1997.

Arlin ML. The periodontal examination and consultation, the diagnostic components. *Oral Health* 76(1):37-42, 1986.

Armitage GC. *Biologic Basis of Periodontal Maintenance Therapy.* Praxis Publishing Co., San Fransisco, 1984.

Ascorbate Action. R.J. Cameron, Winnipeg, MB Canada, 1 (1-6).

Balch JF Jr, Balch PA. *Nutritional Outline for the Professional,*1983.

Bartz FH. *The Key to Good Health Vitamin C.* Fred H. Bartz, Oak Park, 1971.

Becker RO, Selden G. *The Body Electric, Electromagnetism and the Foundation of Life.* William Morrow, New York, 1985.

Benton M. *The Life Science Health System. Part XII.* College of Life Science. Austin, TX.

Berland T. *How to Keep Your Teeth After 30.* Public Affairs Committee, Inc., 1970.

Besford J. *Good Mouthkeeping.* Oxford University Press, London,1984.

The best way to put your money where your mouth is. *Consumer Reports,* March 1984.

Bhaskar S. *Review of Periodontics.* Nov. 5, 1985.

Bland J. *Vitamin C - The Future is Now.* Keats Publishing, New Canaan, CT, 1995.

Bleznakov EG, Hunt GL. *The Miracle Nutrient Coenzyme Q10.* Bantam Books, 1987.

Blond J. *Nutraerobics.* Harper & Row Publishers, San Francisco.

Borell G. *The Peroxide Story.* Echo, Delano, MN, 1986.

Boyd RL. Effects on gingivitis of daily rinsing with 1.5% H_2O_2,*J Clin Periodont* 16:557-562, 1989.

Brotman RH. *Let's Look at your Teeth.* House of Field, Inc., New York.

Cali VM. *The New Lower-Cost Way to End Gum Trouble Without Surgery.* Warner Books, New York, 1982.

Cameron E. *Protocol for the Use of Intraveneous Vitamin C in the Treatment of Cancer.*

Canty LM, Baranowski Z *Colloidal Silver, The Antibiotic Alternative.* The Colloidal Research Foundation, Carmichael, CA, 1994.

Carper J. *Jean Carper's Total Nutrition Guide.* Bantam Books, New York, 1987.

Challem JJ. *Vitamin C Updated.* Keats Publishing, New Canaan, CT, 1983.

Chase R Jr, Keyes PH. Salt, soda and hydrogen peroxide... is it enough? *Florida Dental Journal* 52(2):12-17, 1981.

Cheraskin E, *Vitamin C... Who Needs It?* Arlington Press, Birmingham, 1993.

Cheraskin E, Ringsdorf MW Jr, Sisley EL. *The Vitamin C Connection.* Bantam Books, New York, 1984.

Clinical Signs "Not Enough" in Checking Disease. American Dental Association, 18(4) 1987, 18(11) 1987.

Cobb CM, Rodgers RL, Killow WJ. Ultrastructural examination of human periodontal pockets following the use of an oral irrigation device in vivo. *J Periodont* 59(3), 1988.

Colloidal Silver Handbook, The. The Silver Education Coalition. Salt Lake City.

Colliodal Silver, The Amazing Alternative to Antibiotics. The Association For Advanced Colloid Research, 1994.

Cranin AN. *Dental Health.* Stein and Day, New York, 1971.

Davis A. *Let's Get Well.* Signet, New York, 1972.

Dello Russo NM. The post-prophylaxis periodontal abscess: etiology and treatment. *The International Journal of periodontics and restorative dentistry* 1:29-42, 1985.

Denholtz M, Denholtz E. *How to Save Your Teeth and Your Money.* Van Nostrand Reinhold Co., New York, 1977.

Donsbach K. *What You Always Wanted to Know About Hydrogen Peroxide.* 1987.

Fellman B. A Nutritional Plan for Terrific Teeth. *Prevention,* Dec. 1981.

Fels H. Fluoridation-Health Hoax? *East West,* Oct. 1989.

French CK, et al. DNA probe detection of periodontal pathogens. *Oral Microbiol Immunol* 1:58-62, 1986.

Gargiulo AW, Gargiulo AV. *Detection of Periodontal Disease: Parameters to Asses Periodontal Disease Activity.*

Genco RJ. Highlights of the conference and perspectives for the future. *J Periodont Res* 22:164-171, 1987.

Genco RJ, Zambon JJ. Clinical microbiology in the diagnosis and treatment of periodontal disease. *Journal of American College of Dentists* 56(4):19-27, 1989.

Genco RJ, Zambon JJ, Christersson LA. Use and interpretation of microbiological essays in periodontal diseases. *Oral microbiol and immunol* 1:73-79, 1986.

Gilpin JL. Xerostomia. A Review for Dental Hygienists. *Journal of Dental Hygiene,* March-April 1989.

Gold SI. Early origins of hydrogen peroxide use in oral hygiene. *J Periodont* 54(4):247, 1983.

Graham J, Odent M. *The Z Factor.* Thorsons Publishing Group. Wellingborough, Northamptonshire, 1986.

Greenstein G. Advance in periodontal disease diagnosis. *The International Journal of Periodontics and Restorative Dentistry* 10(5):351-371, 1990.

Greenstein G. The ability of subgingival irrigation to enhance periodontal health. *Compend Contin Educ Dent* 9(4):327.

Greenwell H, Bissada NF, Stovsky DA. Periodontics in general practice: Perspectives on surgical therapy. *Gen Dent* 37(3):228-233, 1989.

Greenwell H, Bissada NF, Wittwer JW. Periodontics in general practice: Perspectives on periodontal diagnosis. *JADA* 119:537-541, Oct. 1989.

Greenwell H, Stovsky DA, Bissada NF. Periodontics in general practice: perspectives on nonsurgical therapy. *JADA* 115:591-595, Oct. 1987.

Grotz W. *1982-1988. 35% Food Grade Hydrogen Peroxide Therapy.*

Guy H. *You Are Your Own Dentist.* Henry Guy DDS, 1985.

Hazard S. Some Early Ideas About Healthful Living. *Healthful Living,* Nov. 1983.

Heaney RP, Barger-Lux MJ. *Calcium and Common Sense.* Doubleday,New York, 1988.

Hill J. *Understanding Gum Disease.* Berkshire Press. West Cornwall, CT, 1984.

Hill WR, Pillsbury DM. *Argyria, The Pharmacology of Silver.* The Williams and Wilkens Co., Baltimore, 1939.

Himber J. *The Complete Family Guide to Dental Health.* McGraw-Hill Book Co, New York, 1977.

Hoag PM, Pawlack EA. *Essentials of Periodontics.* The C.V. Mosby Company, St. Louis, 1990.

Hoffman JM. *The Missing Link.*

The Holistic Dental Digest and *The Once Daily Networker.* The Once Daily Inc., New York, 1985-1993.

Hoogendoorn H, Piessens JP, Scholtes W, Stoddard LA. Hypothiocyanite Ion; the inhibitor formed by the system lactoperoxidase - thiocyanate hydrogen peroxide, *Caries Res* 11:77-84, 1977.

Huggins HA. Preventing Gingivitis Nutritionally. *Let's Live,* Aug. 1989.

Huggins HA. The Significance of Nutrition in Preventive Dentistry. *Let's Live,* March 1989.

Jirgensons B, Straumanis ME. *A Short Textbook of Colloid Chemistry.* The Macmillan Co., New York, 1962.

Jones WHS. Philosophy and Medicine in Ancient Greece. *Ares Publishers Inc.,* Chicago, 1979.

Kaldahl WB, Kalkwarf KL, Patil KD, et al. Evaluation of four modalities of periodontal therapy. *J Periodont* 59(12), 1988.

Kazakos GM. *A light and scanning electron microscopy. Study of the soft tissue change associated with subgingival placement of monolithic tetracycline-impregnated fibers.* M.S. Thesis, University of Missouri, Kansas City, 1989.

Kennedy D. The New Oral Tradition. *Solstice,* Issue #34, Dec.1988-Jan. 1989.

Kenyon C. *How to Avoid Rip-offs at the Dentist.* Sovereign Books, New York, 1979.

Keyes PH, Rams TE. A rationale for management of periodontal diseases: Rapid identification of microbiol therapeutic targets with phase-contrast microscopy. *JADA* 106(6):803-812, 1983.

Kimbrough H, Martin P. Homeopathy in Dental Practice. *Let's Live,* July 1989.

Langer S. *Dental Problems.* Keats Publishing, New Canaan, CT, 1984.

LeBeau C. *Hydrogen Peroxide Therapy.* Pin, Hales Corners, WI, 1987.

Lee WH. *Coenzyme Q-10.* Keats Publishing, New Canaan, CT, 1987.

Leggott PJ, Robertson PB, Rothman DL, Murray PA, Jacob RA. Response of lingual ascorbic acid test and salivary ascorbate levels to changes in ascorbic acid intake. *J Dent Res* 65(2):131-134, Feb. 1986.

Lesser M. *Nutrition and Vitamin Therapy.* Grove Press, New York, 1980.

Levine RA. A patient-centered periodontal program for the 1990's,Part II. *Compend Contin Educ Dent* 11(5):274-284, 1990.

The Linus Pauling Institute of Science and Medicine Newsletter. Palo Alti, CA, 1988-1993.

Listgarten MA. A perspective on periodontal diagnosis. *Journal of Chemical Periodontology,* 13(3):175-180, 1986.

Livacari GL. *A Homecare Program for the Prevention of Gum Disease.* Chicago, 1990.

Lloyd GER, Chadwick J, Mann WN. Hippocratic Writings. *Penguin Books,* New York, 1983.

Loe H. Periodontology in the past 20 years. *Periodontology TO-DAY,* Oct. 1986.

Low SB, Ciancio SG. Reviewing nonsurgical periodontal therapy. *JADA* 121:467-470, Oct. 1990.

Lucas L. Vitamin C and Other Good Things for Your Gums. *Prevention,* Aug. 1980.

Marshall HB. *How to Save Your Teeth.* Everest House Publishers. New York, 1980.

Mayo WL. Australia's Amazing Tea Tree Oil. *Let's Live,* Sept. 1991.

McCabe E. *Oxygen Therapies.* Energy Publications, Morrisville, NY, 1988.

MacFadden B. *Home Health Manual.* MacFadden Book Company, Inc., New York, 1930.

McGuire T. *The Tooth Trip.* Random House, New York, 1980.

Mazer E. Perfect teeth? Why not? *Prevention,* Nov. 1983.

The Merck Manual of Diagnosis and Therapy. Merck Sharp & Dohme Research Laboratories, 1982.

Miller FD. *Healthy Teeth Through Proper Nutrition.* Arco Publishing, New York, 1978.

Nara RO, Mariner SA. *How to Become Dentally Self-Sufficient.* Oramedics International Press, Houghton, MI.

National Institute of Dental Health Fact Sheet. U.S. Dept. of Health and Human Services.

Newbold HL. *Vitamin C Against Cancer.* Stein and Day Publishers,New York, 1979.

Newbrun E, Hoover CI, Ryder MI. Bacterial action of bicarbonate ion on selected periodontal pathogenic microorganisms. *J Periodontol* 55(11):658-667, 1989.

Newman HN. *Dental Plaque.* Charles C Thomas-Publisher. Springfield, IL, 1980.

New Ways to Save Your Teeth? *Consumer Reports*, Aug. 1989.

Nguyen NT, De Roulf P. *Your Mouth, Oral Care for All Ages.* Chilton Book Co, Radnor, PA, 1979.

Nonsurgical antibacterial approaches to periodontal treatment. *JADA* 116:23-32, 1988.

Nonsurgical Treatment of Gum Disease. Healthfacts, New York, 13(111) Aug. 1988.

Nutri-Healthdata. World Research Foundation. Sherman Oaks, CA, 1987.

Olsen CB. *Australian Tea Tree Oil.* Kali Press.

Page ME, Abrams HL Jr. *Your Body is Your Best Doctor!* Keats Publishing, New Canaan, CT, 1972.

Pauling L. *How to Live Longer and Feel Better.* W.H. Freeman & Co., New York, 1986.

Pauling L. *Vitamin C. The Common Cold and the Flu.* W.H. Freeman & Co., San Francisco, 1976.

"Paul Revere". *Dentistry and Its Victims.* St. Martin's Press, New York.

PDA Network News. The People's Dental Association, 1985-1986.

Pearlman B. Starting your own periodontics program. *Dental Outlook* 10(1):1-10, 1984.

Pekkanen J. Do These Dentists Do too Much? *Readers Digest*, Oct.1986.

Periodontal Disease. The Health Base, a service of Prevention magazine.

Periodontal Disease. Healthfacts, New York, 11(83), April 1986.

Phillips JE. *Acquiring and Maintaining Oral Health.* JE Phillips, 1985.

Pichel M, Curtis N. *Have Healthy Teeth and Gums.* Javelin Books, Poole, Dorset, 1986.

Prevention, Rodale Press, Emous, PA, 1975 to 1993.

Price WA. *Nutrition and Physical Degeneration.* The American Academy of Applied Nutrition, Los Angeles, 1939.

Rams TE, Keyes PH, Wright WE, Howard SA. Long-term effects of microbiologically modulated periodontal therapy on advanced adult periodontitis. *JADA* 111:429-441, Sept. 1985.

Rams TE, Keyes PH. Nonsurgical management of rapidly progressive periodontitis. *Gen Dent* 34(1):54-59, 1986.

A review for Xerostomia. American Dental Hygienists Association, *Journal of Dental Hygiene* March-April 1989.

Ring ME. *Dentistry: An Illustrated History, 1985.*

Roach M. Beating Bad Breath. *Hippocrates,* July-August 1989.

Rodale R. Taking Control of Your Teeth and Gums. *Prevention*, June 1983.

Rosenbaum ME. Vitamin C, New and Improved. The Promise of Ester-C. *Health World,* July-August 1989.

Rylander H. Changing concepts of periodontal treatment: surgical and nonsurgical. *Internation Dental Journal* 38(3):163-169, 1988.

Sheffrey S. *Vitamin C - The Pros and Cons.* Prion Books, Ann Arbor, 1991.

Shelton HM. *Superior Nutrition.* Willow Publishing Inc., San Antonio, 1982.

Shelton HM. *The Hygienic System.* Dr. Shelton Health School, San Antonio, 1975.

Soaring Bear. *Dental Self Help.* Soaring Bear, Tucson, AZ, 1983.

Socransky SS. Rationale for the development of diagnostic tests for destructive periodontal disease. *Abstract and audio cassette lecture.*

Stone I. *The Healing Factor "Vitamin C" Against Disease.* Grosset and Dunlap, New York, 1972.

Stults VJ, Sapiro KTS, Clemens RA, Adams GS. Evaluation of a lingual test for vitamin C status. *Journal of Oral Medicine* 42(4):229-232, 1987.

Takata T, Donath K. The mechanism of pocket formation. A light microscopic study on undecalcified human material. *J Periodont* 59(4): 215-221, 1988.

Thomson B. Do Oxygen Therapies Work? *East West*, Sept. 1989.

Toothpastes. *Consumer Reports*, March 1986.

Valentine RL. A Rationale for periodontal therapy in the Keyes era. *J Western Soc Periodont/Periodont Abs* 33(1):5-22,1985.

Watt DL. *Second Opinion, Taking the Bite Out of Dentistry*, 1989.

Wennstrom J, Lindhe J. Effect of hydrogen peroxide on developing plaque and gingivitis in man. *J Clin Periodontol* 6:115-130, 1979.

Wennstrom JL, Heijl L, Dahlen G, Grondahl K. Periodic subgingival antimicrobial irrigation of periodontal pockets. *J Clin Periodontol* 14(9):541-550, 1987.

When should we use X-rays? *Health Science*, Jan.-Feb. 1991.

Williams RJ. *Nutrition Against Disease.* Pitman Publishing Corp., New York.

Williard T. *Feeling Good with Natural Remedies.* Wild Rose College of Natural Healing, Calgary, Alberta.

Winters J. *Breakthrough.* Winters, 1986.

Wolner SZ. Brushing off Periodontal Disease. *Diabetes Self- Management*, Aug. 1987.

Wolner SZ. Mouthwash Alert. *Bruce Jenner's Better Health and Living*, Dec. 1985.

Yiamouyiannis J. *Fluoride: The Aging Factor.* Delaware,Ohio Health Action Press, 1983.

INDEX